Peter Selby is Professor of Cancer Medicine at the University of Leeds and a consultant physician at St James's University Hospital, Leeds, and previously at the Royal Marsden Hospital in London. Born in 1950 in Gloucestershire, he graduated in science from Cambridge University in 1971 and in medicine in 1974. He trained in oncology and cancer research in London and Toronto and became a professor in Leeds in 1988. He is vice-chairman of the Cellular and Molecular Medicine Research Board of the Medical Research Council, president of the British Oncological Association and director of the Imperial Cancer Research Fund Cancer Medicine Research Unit at Leeds; he chairs the Regional Research Committee of Yorkshire Health and the Cancer Research Campaign Committee on Education and Psychological Medicine. He is married with two young children.

Sally Wheeler is Personnel Director at the University of Leeds. Born in Zambia in 1936, she was educated in Africa and at the University of Bristol, where she took a degree in psychology and philosophy. She returned to Africa and enjoyed a variety of careers – as university lecturer, school teacher, librarian, research consultant and journalist – before settling in Britain and becoming a university administrator in 1975. She has four adult children. She was successfully treated for cancer in 1977.

SALLY WHEELER AND PETER SELBY

CONFRONTING CANCER

CAUSE AND PREVENTION

PENGUIN BOOKS

PENGUIN BOOKS

Published by the Penguin Group
Penguin Books Ltd, 27 Wrights Lane, London W8 5TZ, England
Penguin Books USA Inc., 375 Hudson Street, New York, New York 10014, USA
Penguin Books Australia Ltd, Ringwood, Victoria, Australia
Penguin Books Canada Ltd, 10 Alcorn Avenue, Toronto, Ontario, Canada M4V 3B2
Penguin Books (NZ) Ltd, 182–190 Wairau Road, Auckland 10, New Zealand

Penguin Books Ltd, Registered Offices: Harmondsworth, Middlesex, England

First published 1993
1 3 5 7 9 10 8 6 4 2

Typeset by Datix International Limited, Bungay, Suffolk
Printed in England by Clays Ltd, St Ives plc

Contents

List of Figures   vii
Foreword by Sir Walter Bodmer, PhD, FRCPath,
    FRS   ix
Preface   xi
Acknowledgements   xiii

1   Introduction   1
2   What is Cancer?   8
3   The Causes of Cancer   26
4   Smoking and Cancer   63
5   Diet and Cancer   85
6   Skin, Sunlight and Melanoma   121
7   Radiation and Cancer   139
8   Sex, Hormones and Reproduction   152
9   Cancer, the Workplace and Environmental Pollution   166
10   Inherited Cancer – the New Genetics   180
11   The Mind, Society and Cancer   189
12   Cancer and Infections – the Anti-cancer Vaccination?   197
13   Screening for Cancer   203
14   How Much Cancer is Preventable?   221
15   Practical Advice   232
16   What Does the Future Hold?   234
17   Government, Individuals and the National Health
    Service   240

Index   243

List of Figures

1   Curability of cancer
2   The dividing helix
3   DNA codes for RNA
4   The development of a cancer cell
5   Signals for growth control
6   Estimated incidence and mortality for all cancer except skin cancer (a) in men (b) in women
7   Map of the risk of lung cancer in men aged under forty-five years in England and Wales, 1968–81, by county of residence
8   Map of mortality from cancer of the lung in men
9   Map of mortality from cancer of the breast in women
10 Map of mortality from cancer of the oesophagus in men
11 Smoking and lung cancer
12 Dietary fat and breast cancer
13 Link between carotene intake, cigarette smoking and lung cancer
14 The protective effect of vitamin A related materials against second cancers in the head and neck
15 Risk of getting a malignant melanoma (a) in the United States (b) in Scotland
16 Thin melanomas in Australia
17 The natural history of a cancer
18 (a) Screening works (b) Screening fails (c) Screening cannot help
19 Trends in the annual age-adjusted incidence rates of invasive carcinoma of the cervix

20 Percentage of cancer deaths by cause
21 Incidence in Yorkshire of lung cancer in males
22 Trends in mortality from cancer in men aged from twenty to forty-four across Europe

Foreword

Sir Walter Bodmer, PhD, FRCPath, FRS
Director General, Imperial Cancer Research Fund

Cancer is a word that used to be a taboo in everyday discussion but, fortunately, that attitude has changed substantially. Many people, however, still think that cancer is an almost inevitable death sentence and are not aware of the enormous extent to which cancer can actually now be cured. But the most important message surely must be to aim for prevention of cancer in the first place. Many lines of evidence indicate that most cancers have an environmental basis that should ultimately be explainable. If that is the case, it should be possible to recommend lifestyles that lead to the avoidance of most cancers. So far, the one direct and overwhelming message is that smoking cigarettes is a cause of 30 per cent of all cancers in this country, and such cancers should clearly be avoidable. Diet comes next in importance, but we do not yet know precisely what components matter most. Beyond that, there are the effects of sunlight on melanomas and other skin cancers, the effects of avoidable radiation, of chemicals in the environment, of sexual behaviour, of viruses and the contribution that can be made by early detection. All of these questions are discussed in a balanced and effective way in this outstandingly clear book by Sally Wheeler and Peter Selby. Starting from a clear description of the nature of cancer, its incidence and the excitement that modern research is providing in its basic understanding, the authors take us step by step through those factors that we now know to be causes, ending up with a clear message as to the simple measures that can now be taken towards preventing much cancer. The message is a clear and important one for all, and there is no doubt that this book can and should make a major contribution to helping us avoid all the cancers that can be prevented on the basis of our present knowledge.

Preface

Cancer specialists and cancer research workers usually try to avoid discussing their subject at parties. The subject is a sensitive one for all too many people and never makes for light-hearted conversation. This book, however, arises from one such conversation. A comment that modest alterations in our lifestyles would bring about a much larger reduction in cancer deaths than any of the recent advances in therapy was met with some doubt. Fellow guests observed that it was difficult to distinguish between the facts about cancer and claims made by people with little evidence for their strong opinions.

This book is an attempt to remove some of the doubts. We now have a lot of information about the causes and prevention of cancer and some things can be said with certainty. The link between smoking and cancer is a good example of this. The value of screening with cervical smear tests is another. In addition, we can identify some factors which may well be linked to cancer in a complex way but which cannot yet finally be proved to have a connection. The links between fat intake and breast cancer would come into this category. We may make some recommendations based on probabilities because it will be decades before all of the answers are known for certain. Finally, there are a number of highly uncertain claims, particularly about diet and other factors in the environment, and these have to be handled very cautiously at present.

Prevention depends on an understanding of *cause*, and the account which we give of the extent of our understanding necessarily takes us into the realm of science. We have not, however, assumed any deep scientific knowledge on the part of the reader and have tried to explain those scientific terms which we cannot avoid.

This book is the result of a joint effort between someone with a long-standing professional interest in cancer research and cancer care and someone without professional expertise in the subject but who once had the disease. Through this collaboration we have sought to produce a book which is accurate and informed, critical and cautious, but also intelligible to the man and woman in the street. We hope that our broad survey of the present state of our knowledge will also prove valuable to those in the field of health care whose work requires that they have some understanding of the nature and causes of cancer. We should be delighted if our readership were to include young people, since they are in the best position to reduce the occurrence of certain kinds of cancer in the future.

In our society, the very word 'cancer' is invested with a fear that is at odds with our growing understanding of the nature of the diseases and their cause. Readers may find it difficult to accept in a cool and dispassionate frame of mind some of the facts which we put forward. Some potential readers will avoid the book simply because they are too frightened even to think about the subject. Others with habits such as smoking, which involve known risks, would rather not be reminded of the odds. The authors are convinced that knowledge undermines the power of a disease to terrorize. We seek through this book to spread such knowledge as we have and to help those who wish to use the present state of our understanding to minimize some of the hazards now known to be associated with the development of cancer. Cancer may be a conversation-stopper at parties but it is most emphatically not a mysterious scourge against which we are defenceless!

Acknowledgements

Warm thanks go to the following professional colleagues who have given their time to read through chapters and give us most helpful comments and corrections:

Professor Ray Cartwright, Leukaemia Research Fund Professor of Cancer Epidemiology, University of Leeds; Professor Jocelyn Chamberlain, Director, Cancer Screening Evaluation Unit, Royal Marsden Hospital, London; Professor Clair Chilvers, Professor of Epidemiology, University of Nottingham; Dr Steven Greer, Consultant in Psychological Medicine, Royal Marsden Hospital, London; Dr Bob Haward, Regional Director of Public Health Medicine, Yorkshire Health; Ms Jean King, Head of Education, Cancer Research Campaign, London; Professor Richard Lilford, Professor of Obstetrics and Gynaecology, University of Leeds; Professor Rona MacKie, Professor of Dermatology, University of Glasgow; Professor Gerald Richards, Professor of Public Health Medicine, University of Leeds; Dr Gwen Turner, Associate Specialist in Clinical Genetics, Leeds General Infirmary.

The authors nevertheless take full responsibility for the contents of the book.

The manuscript was prepared with great skill, energy and patience by Nicole Goldman, to whom we are most grateful.

Last but not least we should like to thank our families and friends, who encouraged us to write this book and showed great tolerance when we neglected them in the process.

I

Introduction

The statistics on cancer do not make for pleasant reading, but if we are to take a cool and objective look at this disease, we had better confront them. Cancer intrudes on many individual lives and has a major impact on the national life of many countries. One in three people will develop a cancer and about one in four will die of cancer. These statistics must be viewed against the fact that we can successfully treat and have almost eliminated a number of other diseases. Life expectancy has increased in the richer parts of the world. This will lead to more cancer cases because the disease is commoner in older people. The human and economic cost of the incidence of cancer is enormous and defies accurate assessment. A vast range of cancer treatment services, from surgery to terminal care, are provided by the health-care systems of developed countries. Sometimes these treatments produce cures and sometimes they fail. They are always expensive. A recent conservative estimate by the government of the cost of hospital care for cancer in the United Kingdom was £2 billion each year. The cost in terms of the suffering for patients and their families cannot be gauged. Over £100 million is spent annually on cancer research in the United Kingdom, mainly from charitable donations, and large sums are spent by government and international agencies throughout the world on registering, studying and analysing the information about cancer patients.

Above and beyond these daunting statistics lies the very special fear that cancer generates in people's minds. Even though expert modern cancer care can sometimes cure and almost always control the major symptoms of the disease, many people still fear cancer more than the other common serious and life-threatening diseases of our times. They see it as an especially 'sneaky' disease, often lurking unrecognized and symptomless until discovered by accident. They may view cancer with despair as 'the enemy within' – an uninvited attack by the body on itself. They use euphemisms like 'the big C', as if uttering the very word 'cancer' will render them vulnerable. Misplaced fears of acquiring cancer by contact with cancer patients still persist and it is not unknown for cancer patients to feel lonely, guilty or inadequate (emotions which are not usually associated with other common diseases).

Health-care professionals themselves are not immune from emotional responses to this disease. For doctors, cancer generates a number of challenges. Some of the surgeon's largest and most complex operations will be carried out on cancer patients. For the physician, cancer presents some of the most difficult diagnoses and testing questions about appropriate treatment. Experts in diagnostic procedures in the laboratory or in the reading of diagnostic X-rays and scans are faced with the challenge of detecting a cancer when it is early and treatable. It is hardly surprising that cancer care can generate the most tremendous satisfaction for the doctor who is successful in curing or controlling the disease. Nor should it surprise anyone that the most dismal sensations of frustration and failure are sometimes felt by doctors when they confront the results of cancer care. The care of cancer patients may present particular challenges to nurses too, placing heavy demands upon their dedication. Those who manage health care are under constant pressure to find more resources for cancer treatment and care against competing demands on their limited budgets. The very success of modern medical science in understanding, curing or eliminating other diseases which were once viewed with horror raises the emotional stakes for those involved in cancer research and therapy.

The steady stream of newspaper articles and radio and television programmes about possible causes of cancer is undoubtedly intended to inform the public and give hope that this disease will one day be well enough understood to be completely curable. Cancer is 'news'. Unfortunately, the news is often presented with morbid glamour. It can give an impression of cancer as some kind of scourge which has been visited upon us or which we have brought on ourselves. New cancer hazards are presented to us at every turn – in our choice of food, in the nature of our occupations, in the location of our homes, in our technological advances and in the simple act of drinking water from a tap – and we may be left feeling guilty, bewildered or helpless. This book is an attempt to put the disease into perspective. We shall examine the extent of cancer, evaluate the state of our knowledge about its causes and assess the extent to which this knowledge can be used to prevent cancer. We will explain how knowledge about the causes of cancer is accumulated and discuss some of the difficulties always found in these studies. Against this background, we shall try to provide practical guidance about the avoidance of cancer, indicating what can be recommended with certainty, what can be done reasonably in the state of present knowledge and, finally, which other ideas have to be regarded as purely speculative at present.

The message about the prevention of cancer can now be an optimistic one in many important respects. Not only do we know what needs to be done but we also have evidence that these measures can be successful in reducing the frequency of many common cancers. We will review the present trends in cancer occurrence in some detail and demonstrate that the clear fall in the rates for many common cancers in younger people in many countries bodes well for the future. We must acknowledge that there are also areas of grave concern, where the evidence suggests either no decrease or even an increase for some cancers. These perhaps require particular attention because simple measures might well make a difference and avoid further increases.

This book cannot, by its very nature, be a comprehensive guide to the diagnosis and treatment of all kinds of cancer, but it would not be complete without at least general comments on the areas where diagnosis and treatment have generated major changes and on where further efforts are likely to be successful. Early diagnosis by screening is a very topical subject, but the success of screening remains restricted to a few types of cancer at present. Cancer treatment by surgery, radiotherapy, chemotherapy and, more recently, biological therapy is having an impact (Figure 1), and great improvements in outlook have been achieved with some cancers over the last two decades. Great strides are being made in the biological sciences and we need to consider whether these are likely to generate major advances in cancer treatment in the near future.

At this point we should give some information about cancer treatment. It is important for people to realize that cancer is often cured. Between one third and one half of all cancer patients have successful treatments and subsequently live almost entirely normal lives. Some common cancers, such as those arising in the large bowel (colon and rectum), some breast cancers, kidney cancers and bladder cancers, are, when diagnosed early, localized to their primary site. Such cancers can be removed by an operation and these operations are curative. Thousands of people with these cancers are cured every year. Surgery has not produced a much greater proportion of cures in the last few years but surgeons are becoming more skilful at minimizing the damaging effects of their operations. This means that it is often possible to remove a cancer without leaving large scars or without removing a whole organ. Perhaps the greatest benefits have come from conservative breast cancer surgery, leaving the breast intact after surgery

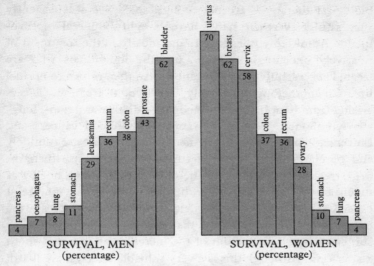

Figure 1 Curability of cancer.

This figure shows the percentage of people with each of the commoner cancers who can be expected to be alive five years after the diagnosis. For many cancers, if someone is alive and well and free of their disease after five years they are probably cured. Unfortunately, this is not true for all cancers, so these percentages should only be taken as general guidelines describing the proportion of people who are cured with each cancer. Perhaps the most notable point is that the commonest cancer, cancer of the lung, has a very poor chance of cure. (Prepared from data provided by the Cancer Research Campaign.)

and perhaps following up with additional treatment like radiotherapy or chemotherapy to try to ensure cure. Surgery is a successful treatment for many people. Radiotherapy is capable of curing some localized cancers – notably those arising in the head and neck and some gynaecological cancers. Although less successful than surgery, it is still a very useful treatment for many people. Treatments with drugs – chemotherapy and biological therapy – are newer and, so far, less consistently successful. Nevertheless, they have brought about real improvements. Admittedly, these are found mostly in the treatment of relatively uncommon cancers, but the individuals who are treated successfully for these cancers can then return to normal life. Chemotherapy is notably effective in treating cancers arising from lymph glands – Hodgkin's disease and non-Hodgkin lymphomas – leukaemias, many childhood cancers and cancers arising in the testes in men. Many of these are routinely and regularly cured by drug treatment. In other situations, drug treatment can increase the cure rate, although not by as much as we would like. The best example is that of breast cancer, where careful use of drug treatment can increase the cure rate significantly above that which can be obtained by surgery alone. The amount of the increase varies but is about 10 per cent. Although this is a very valuable effect, there is still room for great improvement.

Probably the best examples of progress by drug treatment are in the treatment of testicular cancers in young men and the treatment of cancer in children.

Cancer in the testis is not common, but it is the commonest form of cancer in men aged between twenty and thirty-four in the United Kingdom and there are about one thousand new cases every year. A man has only a 1 in 480 chance of developing a testicular cancer at some time in his life so the odds in his favour are pretty high.

Once testicular cancer has spread to the rest of the body (secondary spread or metastasis) it can only be treated effectively with drugs. Before 1970 there was no successful drug treatment and everybody who developed secondary spread from a testicular cancer died of the disease. In the early 1970s, some drugs were used successfully for the first time and between 10 and 20 per cent of patients were cured. There were dramatic improvements in drug treatment during the 1970s with the introduction, in particular, of a new group of drugs based on the metal platinum. The platinum drugs were so successful that, by the end of the 1970s, 80 per cent of young men with widespread testicular cancer were cured. Now the results have improved even further and over 90 per cent of patients are cured. This is a major advance.

Cancers in children are very rare but until effective drug treatments were introduced they were often fatal because the diseases tend to be widespread. However, many (sadly, not all) children's cancers have now yielded to effective drug treatment and over half are cured. This has transformed the outlook for children with cancer and in many cases the emphasis can now be on ensuring the best quality of life for the survivors as they grow up.

We are obviously seeking to introduce such improvements in the prospects for those with other cancers but, so far, drug treatments are not having such a dramatic effect in common cancers. Sadly, some of the commonest cancers, such as lung cancer in particular, are those that are least curable. Improved treatments for cancer are the subject of intensive research. However, treatment is not the subject of this book – we have set out to discuss cause and prevention.

2

What is Cancer?

The human body, like most living organisms, is assembled from millions and millions of individual cells. The cells are the building bricks of the body, making up the skin, blood and every functioning part. We start life as a single cell, which is brought about by the fertilization of a single egg by a single sperm. Each cell multiplies by dividing into two cells (called 'daughter' cells), and the resulting collection of cells develops into the unborn child. Growth into adult life requires further huge multiplication of cells, a process known as *cellular proliferation*. Once we reach adult life certain parts of our bodies require continuous repair and renewal. We are continuously shedding our skin, the lining of our intestines and the lining of our lungs and bladders; and, as these are shed, the cells in these organs are replaced by further proliferation. Cellular proliferation is therefore a basic process for maintaining life and health.

The proliferation of cells is linked to a process by which cells in different parts of the body develop different functions. Heart cells have to contract to push blood around the body, liver cells become chemical factories altering the content of our diet to turn it into the essential nutrition for all parts of the body. Cells which line the gut or cover the skin are developed specially for these purposes. The process by which cells develop different functions is called *differentiation*.

Cancer is a disease in which cellular proliferation and differentiation become disordered. The problem with cancer cells is that they continue to proliferate when they should not. This means that too many cells accumulate and this is how tumours are formed (the word tumour comes from the Latin word for a swelling); the accumulation of too many cells as a consequence of proliferation results in tumour masses in the affected part of the body. In addition to exhibiting disordered proliferation, the cancer cell usually fails to behave in the correct way for a cell in a particular location. It lacks correct differentiation. This means that it will look abnormal through a microscope and will behave abnormally, often manufacturing the wrong substances or failing to manufacture the substances that it should be making.

So if cancer is the result of a disorder of the way cells multiply and the way they function, how does it cause the extensive damage that we associate with this disease? Every medical student is taught that there are three essential character-istics of a cancer. These are *growth*, *invasion* and *spread*.

The process of *growth* of a cancer is easy to understand. We have already explained that the controls that normally act on the multiplication of cells are deranged and that excessive numbers of cells accumulate. Sometimes, the multiplication of cells occurs very rapidly but, equally often, the process may not be particularly rapid but may simply continue when it should be switched off. Either way, the result will be an uncontrolled growth of cells within the organ affected. With lung cancer, such a growth will be seen as a shadow on a chest X-ray. For breast cancer, a lump will appear in the breast. For a cancer occurring in the intestines, the lump will not be visible unless special X-rays or scans are used, but it will usually alter the function of the bowel or tend to obstruct it, a process which can produce pain. Sometimes these lumps may bleed, which is why bleeding is a common symptom leading to the diagnosis of cancer in many sites. The process of growth of the cancer is in itself dangerous. For instance, large cancers within the lung will interfere with the function of the lungs and sometimes, when cancers occur in particularly vital situations like the brain, the presence of quite a small growth is capable of causing catastrophic damage. However, growths can often be removed and it is the other features of the cancer which represent the greatest challenges to effective treatment.

Invasion means that instead of remaining contained within its own area of the body the cancer is capable of extending outside this area. A cancer of the lungs is capable of growing into other sites in the chest. A cancer in the intestine is capable of growing through the wall of the intestine and sticking to other organs. This process of invasion may carry the cancer beyond the realm of a single surgical operation and prevent a surgeon from carrying out an operation that might lead to a cure. If extensive invasion has occurred, successful curative surgery is usually not possible.

The final feature of a cancer, which is the one that makes it so difficult to cure in so many cases, is its ability to *spread* to distant sites of the body. This process is called metastasis and metastasis occurs by the spread of cancer cells through the fluid circulations of the body, either tissue fluids called lymph or in the bloodstream. Once a cancer has spread in this way it cannot usually be cured by an operation because so many different sites within the body will be involved. In these situations the potential for cure rests upon the much less fully developed treatments with drugs of either a chemical or biological kind.

Growth, invasion and spread do not occur to the same extent in all cancers. Cancers that arise in different organs of the body have very different patterns of spread and for each individual site from which a cancer can originate there will be a different chance of spread. For instance, lung cancers have a very high probability of spread. At the time of their diagnosis about three quarters of patients will have evidence of spread when they are assessed by their doctors and when tests are carried out. Therefore, only about one quarter of lung cancer patients will have any chance of cure as a result of an operation. Spread may have occurred even though it is not detected by the tests. On the other hand, cancers that arise in the brain cause damage by local growth but very rarely spread outside the brain. The chance of spread for the other commoner cancers such as breast, bowel, bladder and gynaecological cancers is intermediate between these two extremes and spread has generally occurred in between one third and two thirds of all the patients who develop the disease.

These statistics allow plans to be made for assessing and treating most patients. However, even when the diagnosis is made, the doctor will be unable to tell an individual patient with certainty what the outcome of his or her cancer is going to be. If there appears to have been no spread of the cancer and it has been completely removed by an operation, cautious optimism will be due in many cases. If, however, after the tests are done and an operation has been carried out, it is discovered that some of the cancer remains, the outcome will depend upon the chance of treating the remaining cancer by means other than surgery. For some cancers, such as Hodgkin's disease or testicular cancer in men, the chances of effecting a cure in these circumstances will remain high.

Even when cures are not achieved, there remains great uncertainty about the outcome for an individual patient. The progression of a cancer varies tremendously between individual patients. Some cancers grow rapidly and others very slowly. In some cases little change may appear over a period of several years whereas in others rapid changes will occur over a few months. Although examination of the cancer in the laboratory can give important guidance, the information obtained in this way is, as yet, not very precise and there will often be a good deal of uncertainty in the information that is given to a patient.

Cancer and the New Biology

The description of cancer given at the beginning of this chapter might have been written in 1950 or 1960. It represents an understanding of how cancer cells behave in terms of what was then known about cellular biology. Very little was understood about what controlled events within cells and determined (among other things) their proliferation and differentiation. Things began to change in 1953 when Francis Crick and James Watson created their now famous model of the structure of DNA, the double helix. Today we can create computer images of DNA – Crick and Watson built models of wire and cardboard!

Chemical substances are made up of molecules. The discovery by Crick and Watson that DNA, a large molecule found in *all* cells, was shaped like two intertwined strands presented the solution to a problem that had puzzled scientists for years.

The DNA molecule is constructed from four types of smaller and simpler molecules, known as bases, strung out along each strand. Some people like to visualize the double helix as a spiral staircase, with the bases as the steps, and this is quite a good way of thinking about it.

Crick and Watson realized that this double-stranded structure could explain how the biological information in a cell could be copied exactly and transmitted to the two new cells which result when a cell divides. Each step of the spiral staircase consists of a pair of bases bonded in the middle and, because the bases do not pair up at random to form 'steps', but always pair up with a complementary base, each strand in the DNA molecule has a sequence of bases that is exactly complementary to the sequence of bases on its partner strand. When a cell divides, the two strands separate so that the DNA is split along its length. Each strand then becomes a blueprint for making a new partner strand with complementary bases, and the biological information in each new pair of strands is identical to that in the original DNA molecule.

What exactly is this biological information? As we see, there are four types of bases (actually representing four different chemical substances designated by the letters A, T, G and C). These can be thought of as a four-letter code, with the sequence in which the bases are strung out along the strands providing a coded message. Different pieces of the same DNA molecule can each have a unique sequence of bases so that each piece carries its own coded message. The number of different possible sequences using a genetic code of four letters is enormous, especially when we consider that a single typical animal cell contains one metre of DNA. This huge potential for different coded messages is the basis of the great variety that we find in the living world and is, of course, the reason why one species is different from another and why each individual is unique.

Genes are made of DNA. They represent a section of DNA which carries enough information in its coded sequence to instruct the cell to make a particular protein. Each protein will then make up a part of the cell's structure or control an aspect of its function. The unique structure and function of each cell will be determined by the genes carried within that cell.

From 1953 to 1970, knowledge was steadily gained about DNA, the genetic code and other complicated chemical substances within the cell, and the new science of molecular biology was born. Progress was steady but quite slow because of the difficulties in unravelling the appropriate parts of the coding system. It became clear that, within the cell itself, the chemically coded message in the DNA is transcribed into a sequence on another substance called RNA. RNA can be thought of as a messenger substance which then carries that information out from the centre of the cell to all other parts of the cell, where it is translated into the protein form. Slowly, the way in which this occurs was being unravelled.

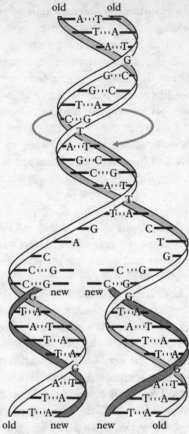

Figure 2 The dividing helix.

Untwisting of DNA strands while it makes a new copy of itself. The strands untwist by rotating about the axis of the unreplicated DNA double helix. A, T, G and C are the bases which make up the code. The 'old' strands of DNA are marked separately from the 'new' ones. One old and one new strand make up each of the two identical new DNA molecules produced by this process.

(From Watson *et al.*, *Molecular Biology of the Gene*, Benjamin/Cummings Publishing Company, California, 1987.)

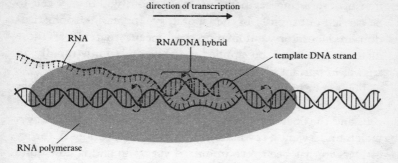

Figure 3 DNA codes for RNA.

The code on the DNA molecule is not directly used to make protein. First a molecule of another substance called RNA is made. This has a sequence of bases which are matched to the DNA. The RNA is the messenger which carries the code out into the cell where proteins are made.

(From Watson *et al.*, *Molecular Biology of the Gene*, Benjamin/Cummings Publishing Company, California, 1987.)

During the 1970s and early 1980s a series of powerful new techniques became available in the laboratories of molecular biologists. Rapid methods for discovering the sequence in DNA were devised. Special chemical substances called enzymes which could be used to cut and rejoin DNA in particular places became available, making it possible to move segments of DNA around almost at will. The means of taking segments of DNA and linking them into the genetic material of microbes followed on from these discoveries. This allowed methods to be devised for growing large quantities of DNA in the laboratory – the process which became known as gene cloning. Powerful techniques became available to probe the DNA of an organism to find the presence of particular sequences and then describe their alterations. Most recently, in the mid-1980s, techniques have been devised which allow the specific amplification of interesting segments of DNA from within any cell to be carried out rapidly in the laboratory. Increasing sophistication in laboratory automation has meant that all of these methods can now be applied reliably and quite rapidly to answer important biological questions.

The application of these powerful laboratory techniques has led to a great explosion of knowledge about the behaviour of cells and the operation and control of the genetic code. Biology, which underwent a revolution through the evolutionary theory of Darwin, has been revolutionized yet again and is now quite commonly referred to as 'the new biology'. This new biology is very different from the description of the behaviour of cells which preceded it and it has of course been applied energetically to studying cancer.

Knowledge about the control of the process of proliferation in cells and differentiation in normal cells has gone hand in hand with knowledge about the disorder of these processes in the cancerous cell. Although the understanding of the behaviour of the cancer cell is far from complete, the application of the new biology has led to a knowledge of cancer far in advance of anything available ten years ago.

THE BASIC UNDERSTANDING OF CANCER

Usually a cancer begins when a single cell within the body undergoes essential changes in its DNA so that the 'switches' which control the processes of proliferation and of differentiation are altered. That cell multiplies by dividing into two cells and the cancer characteristics are transmitted in the DNA to each new 'daughter' cell. Hence each cell that is the product of cellular proliferation has the same version of the genetic code. In this way the characteristics of a cancer are inherited from cell to cell and retained by all the cells within that cancer. Cancer is thus a genetic disease, because the genetic information is passed from cell to cell within the cancer. It is not usually a genetic disease in the sense that its occurrence is passed from parents to their children, although rare examples of that process will be discussed later in this book.

So what are the essential switches that control how the cell behaves and how are they altered to turn that cell into a cancer cell? By no means all the answers to these questions are yet available. However, the new biology has provided a number of them and yielded glimpses of several more.

The first point to make is that the change into a cancer cell does not occur as a result of an alteration in a single controlling gene. A series of changes, as many as half a dozen, will usually be necessary before the full characteristics of a cancer cell develop. One or two changes may produce an abnormal cell, but without all of those characteristics of growth, invasion and metastasis that we considered in the last section.

In Figure 4 we show a theoretical sequence of events in which changes occur in the genetic material of a normal cell to cause it to begin to grow abnormally. The characteristic of abnormal growth is passed on to 'daughter' cells but does not yet form a cancer. The second change increases the abnormal growth pattern and it may give rise to a lump, but this does not spread and is not yet cancer. A further change occurs and now, as we look down the microscope, the growth appears like a cancer but it is growing slowly and does not spread. After a fourth change the cancer starts to grow more rapidly, but a fifth change is necessary before it has all the features of growth and spread which are the hallmarks of the disease. In no single cancer are all these stages, or the exact number of stages, clear, but for some cancers a great deal of information exists. Two important kinds of gene in which changes occur to promote the development of a cancer have now been discovered and there are many examples of each.

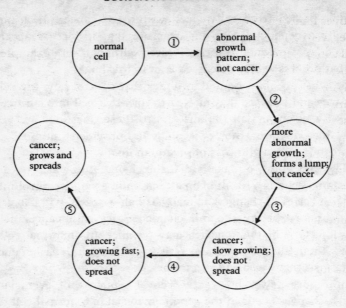

Figure 4 The development of a cancer cell.

Oncogenes

Oncogenes (literally 'cancer genes') were first discovered in the genetic material of viruses that are capable of causing cancers in animals. As the powerful tools of biology were applied to these viruses it became clear that particular genes within them were responsible for altering the cells in the animals that were infected. Although this finding was of great scientific importance, it was initially felt not to be central to the understanding of cancer in humans because viruses are unusual, and often only indirect, causes of cancer in man. The immediate importance of oncogenes in human cancer became clear with the discovery that most of the virus oncogenes had very close relatives that were present in the normal human cell. Moreover, these seem to be very important genes and there are close similarities between these genes in man and in other animals, including mice. When a particular kind of gene occurs in many, many species, this usually means that this type of gene is carrying out a very important function and that it has been conserved for that purpose by each species.

Oncogenes are present in normal cells where they do not cause cancer. In this situation they are called proto-oncogenes. The immediate question was: how do they cause cancer when a virus infects an animal cell? The answer lies in an alteration in the level of activity and the type of activity of such genes. It became clear that although these oncogenes would normally influence the control of cellular proliferation and differentiation in a beneficial and appropriate way, if they were altered so that the sequence of their DNA was slightly different, or if they became overactive because too many copies were present, or if they moved to the wrong part of the genetic material of the cell, then their activity would be disordered. This could result in disordered proliferation and hence contribute to the development of a cancer. Many dozens of oncogenes have now been discovered and it appears very likely that many of them are important in the cause of human cancer. This does not mean that the cancers in humans arise as a result of virus infection. Alterations in these genes can occur as a result of a number of processes and, once they are altered, they can contribute to the formation of the cancer. The virus link with cancer in animals allowed us to discover oncogenes. Overactivity and altered activity of an oncogene is commonly found in many human cancers although the same oncogene may not be altered in all cancers of one organ. Disorder of an oncogene is likely to be one or more of the steps in the creation of a fully fledged cancer and several powerful examples of this are now known for common cancers, including lung cancer and cancer of the bowel.

Each oncogene is now usually given a brief name derived from the virus in which it was first found or from some other feature of its description. The three-letter name is typical and important examples are ras, myc and sis.

We have referred to oncogenes as important elements controlling the behaviour of a cell and, in particular, its proliferation. How do they do this? The answers are still uncertain but many important clues are being revealed and this field of cancer research is one of those developing most rapidly. The functions of different oncogenes may be very different from each other but most of them seem to be involved in the process by which factors control the proliferation of cells.

Thus some oncogenes may provide the genetic information which leads to the manufacture of substances (receptors) on the surface of cells which receive signals instructing that cell to multiply. Some oncogenes may code for the substances within the cell that transmit signals from the surface into the nucleus of the cell where most of the genetic control is occurring. Other oncogenes code for factors which are attached to the nucleus or contained within it which presumably act as the final pathway by which the signals are transmitted into the important control centres. Yet others may actually code for the signalling substances themselves (usually called growth factors). Alterations at any one of these points can result in the wrong message being transferred into the cell telling it to continue proliferating when a normal cell would be switched off, resting and without potential to cause any harm. Alterations in the oncogenes which are responsible for each of these stages in the process of signalling into the cell can therefore contribute to the development of cancer.

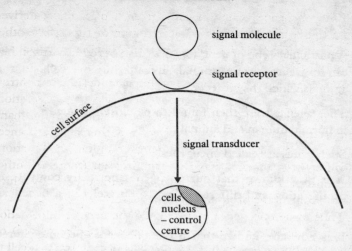

Figure 5 Signals for growth control.

The control signals act to influence the growth of the cell. Signal molecules (often called growth factors) move between cells and attach themselves to receivers or receptors. Different cells in the body have different receptors and this will determine which cells are affected by the signal. Once the signal molecule has bound to the receptor, the signal is conducted (transduced) to the nucleus, where activation occurs using a number of nuclear proteins. If this growth-control process is deranged, then the cells will multiply in an uncontrolled way and this can lead to a cancer. The process may be deranged by alterations in any of the stages. Oncogenes have now been discovered that relate to each of these stages.

The Story of Oncogenes

- A particular type of gene was first discovered in viruses that can cause cancer in animals by altering the cells in the animals which they infect.

- These genes were then found to be closely related to genes in normal human and animal cells.

- Such genes are called oncogenes.

- It is now known that our oncogenes normally control the proliferation and differentiation of our cells in a beneficial way.

- It is now also known that if our oncogenes become altered or disordered, they can contribute to the development of a cancer.

- Alterations in oncogenes can be brought about in a number of ways.

- It is thought likely that at least some of the 'causes of cancer' that we shall identify, such as smoking and radiation, produce cancer by altering oncogenes and other genes.

Tumour Suppressor Genes

Tumour suppressor genes, which determine the development of a cancer in some circumstances, have been discovered more recently than oncogenes. It appears that there are within cells many control elements designed to suppress the development of a cancer. They work by acting as negative controls on the process of cell proliferation and the name 'tumour suppressor gene' is probably the best one, although they are frequently referred to as anti-oncogenes. Tumour suppressor genes are harder to study than oncogenes simply because they act as suppressors. When they are doing their work, there are no cancerous changes to study. A tumour suppressor gene has to be deleted from a cancer cell before the cancer pattern can emerge. Examples of tumour suppressor genes are still relatively few but many more probably remain to be discovered. The best known is a gene that suppresses the development of a rare kind of cancer called retinoblastoma which develops in the eyes of children. This is one of the few cancers that clearly runs in families and it does so because abnormal versions of a particular tumour suppressor gene are inherited from parents by their children. The normal cell contains two copies of the tumour suppressor gene and inheriting a single non-functioning copy from parents is not enough to cause the cancer. The other gene has to be inactivated by a process that occurs after the birth of a child. When both copies are inactive, the cancer develops. In the development of commoner cancers it is unusual for inheritance of an abnormal tumour suppressor gene to be the important mechanism and it is probable that several events must occur after birth before the tumour suppressor genes are fully inactivated. Although these genes were initially discovered as a result of studies carried out in inherited cancers, we now believe that abnormalities in these genes can occur without any inheritance from parents.

The most important tumour suppressor gene known to us so far is probably one called p53, discovered by Professor David Lane at the Imperial Cancer Research Fund in London. It is the gene which is most commonly found to be abnormal in any cancer.

What Causes Malfunction in Oncogenes and Tumour Suppressor Genes?

So far in this chapter we have tried to describe how cancers behave and what the underlying abnormalities in the control processes of their cells are thought to be. It is clear that a number of crucial control elements called genes within the cell have to be altered before it becomes cancerous. What we have not yet said is how these alterations that produce the malfunctioning genes actually occur. A few of the processes that damage the genetic material are well understood, but most can only be described in very general terms. A small number of well-understood examples comes from the study of rare inherited cancers like retinoblastoma. Here it is easy to understand how the inheritance of an abnormal gene from parents can put the child at risk of developing a cancer. There are other examples of inherited cancer patterns. Perhaps the most closely studied is a condition (called familial polyposis coli) in which multiple growths occur in the bowel, many of them turning into cancers. Here again, the inheritance of an abnormal gene from parents puts the patient at risk of developing a cancer. However, we have already said that cancers that clearly run in families represent a small minority. Studying them has given important insights into how cancers develop but cannot tell us what happens for most common cancers where no clear family pattern exists. For these cancers it is likely that the oncogenes and tumour suppressor genes are damaged by factors present in the environment. There are very many chemicals which are known to damage DNA, our genetic material.

Such substances are usually referred to as mutagens (that is *muta*tion-*gen*erating) and when they are capable of causing cancer they are called carcinogens (that is cancer-generating). We believe that exposure of normal cells to damaging substances in the environment produces the changes in oncogenes and tumour suppressor genes that lead on to the development of a cancer. We know that many of the environmental factors which appear to be associated with the development of cancers, each of which will be discussed in some detail in subsequent chapters, are capable of damaging DNA. We do not yet know which environmental factors cause consistent damage to particular oncogenes or whether the damage can (often) occur in many different oncogenes. Perhaps, when we do have this knowledge, the process of preventing cancer will become much simpler to plan and explain. For the time being, the new biology has provided us with an understanding of how cancers grow and what the essential targets for carcinogens are. It has not yet filled in all the gaps to explain step by step the link between cancer-causing substances in the environment and the development of the cancer in the patient.

3

The Causes of Cancer

In the preceding chapter we talked about the nature of cancer and its biology, and described recent discoveries about the process of controlling cancers at the most scientific level. This sort of knowledge is mainly acquired by studies in the laboratory, usually carried out on cancers growing in cultures in plastic or glass dishes under special conditions. These kinds of experiment have provided the dramatic insights described from the new biology and can give important clues about the basic causes of cancer. They tell us how cancer cells grow and what changes are necessary to underpin the development of a cancer. By experiments in which cells in culture are exposed to many agents such as chemicals or radiation we can learn whether these agents are capable under some circumstances of producing cancerous behaviour in target cells. This is experimental science and it is providing us with a powerful tool to enhance our knowledge of the cause of cancer.

Another tool is the observation of the development of cancers in people. Work on the location of cancers and where they spread was mainly carried out in the nineteenth and early twentieth centuries and this process of careful description of what happens to patients, allied to very detailed descriptions of the behaviour of tumours, can still contribute useful knowledge. There remains a role for the doctor or group of doctors who keep meticulous records of the findings with large numbers of patients and the outcome for each and every one of them. This kind of clinical science is important but probably has now contributed most of what it can to our knowledge of cancer.

The third kind of method which helps us understand cancer is the study of the development of cancers in communities and of the links between the cancers seen in communities and other features of life in those communities. This is the science of *epidemiology* and it has, in many ways, been the most revealing of all of the sciences in the study of cancer in this century (although many scientists practising in the laboratory might not share this view). In fact, epidemiology and experimental science and clinical observation are all complementary and, together, can tell us much about the different causes of cancer.

The study of the development of cancers in populations is best illustrated by the link between lung cancer and smoking. This topic merits a chapter in its own right, which will follow later, but the essence of the observations allows us to illustrate how epidemiology can work. As smoking increased in communities in Western Europe and North America so did lung cancer. Within those communities, it seemed to be mainly people who smoked who got lung cancer. Different groups within the society who had different exposure to cigarette smoking had different rates of lung cancer and when particular groups, for instance doctors, reduced their smoking, lo and behold, they got less lung cancer. This is a simple statement of a very complicated story and the net result has been to reveal the single most important known cause of human cancer, cigarette smoke. All of these observations were made by studying the patterns of cancer within communities, although they were extended by experiments in which the important elements of cigarette smoke, particularly tar, were mixed with cells and were shown to be capable of causing cancerous changes. The link between cigarette smoking and lung cancer remains the strongest, clearest and most important link in our entire knowledge of cancer, and the one that presents the greatest potential for winning the war against cancer, at least on that front. In other areas, the links between cancer and lifestyle are much less clear, but they may turn out to be even more important; they certainly require very careful study.

In this chapter we are going to explain how a researcher can work on these problems, how certain of the observations he makes may be very compelling and also what the pitfalls and uncertainties may be. This will provide the basis for discussing each of the important potential causes of cancer, one by one, in ensuing chapters. The values and the limitations of epidemiology are an extremely complex topic and are frequently only well understood by people who are deeply immersed in the subject professionally. Misunderstandings about the strengths and weaknesses of this science have generated considerable confusion among the general public and also among health-care professionals, and it is worth spending some time looking at how the suggestions of epidemiology are studied and evaluated, how they become more certain and how they may well remain unproven despite many years of careful work.

HISTORY

Attempts to unravel the cause of cancer really began in the eighteenth century; perhaps the first milestone was the work of the British surgeon Percival Pott, who in 1775 made the observation that cancer of the scrotum was more common in men who had worked as chimney-sweeps in boyhood. The guess that some substance in soot was causing this cancer on the skin has been borne out by work in the following two centuries. Pott's work also illustrated another important principle. The cancer occurred in men who had worked as chimney-sweeps years before, demonstrating the delayed effect of exposure to some cancer-generating substances. Also in the late eighteenth century, physicians described possible links between snuff-taking and tobacco-smoking and cancers occurring on the nose or on the lip, all of which have been borne out by subsequent observation. The nineteenth century saw further efforts to detect underlying causes for cancers. Physicians and surgeons studied the occurrence of uterine cancers and related these to the reproductive and sexual histories of the patients. They studied the relationship between cancer in the bladder and occupational exposures to chemicals in the dye industry, and they studied the links between industrial exposure of some miners and lung cancer. These valuable studies generated insights into the causes of cancer which will be described in subsequent chapters. The observations were mainly of strong associations. That is to say the risk of suffering from the cancer was greatly enhanced by the particular exposures that were considered. The number of patients included in these studies was usually relatively small and would not have served as a basis for detecting less obvious but important factors in the cause of cancer.

MODERN EPIDEMIOLOGY

This century has seen remarkable growth in the scale and power of the studies carried out by epidemiologists, and in the sophistication and skill with which those studies have been conducted. The growth of the science has been driven by the increased incidence of cancer and the pressure from governments and citizens to have answers, and has been greatly enhanced by the increasing availability of computers and the application of information technology to collecting the facts about cancer in the population.

Epidemiology proceeds on a broad front, integrating knowledge from cancer registries (collections of statistics on officially reported cancer occurrence and mortality), clinical studies and specific studies designed to answer a single question about a possible link between a cancer and a possible causative factor. Answers can often only be deduced by adding together all of these approaches. However, it is easier to describe how epidemiologists work by splitting their activities rather artificially into two kinds: descriptive work and analytical work.

Descriptive Studies

Epidemiologists can gain valuable information from looking at carefully planned descriptions of the patterns of cancer within populations, usually national or regional populations. Because cancers do not occur uniformly in all populations, such studies have provided many important clues about the causes of cancer. Later, we will describe the distributions of different cancers in the European Community to illustrate how much variation can exist even between rather similar countries. Much greater variations exist between countries in different continents and between groups with very different social and economic standing. Some cancers, notably breast cancer, are strongly associated with the pattern of life found in developed societies in Europe and North America. Others, notably cancer of the liver, are found much more frequently in the developing world. Clues can therefore be sought by seeing what factors might be most closely linked to the individual cancers under study. Not only can national, social and economic differences yield information. The incidence of cancer at different ages and in different sexes and different races and at different times in history can yield valuable facts and clues. By studying the pattern of cancers in these groups the epidemiologists will seek to identify factors in the environment or factors in the host (the person with cancer) which put that person at a greater risk of cancer and, when possible, to provide an accurate measurement of the size of that risk.

In any population the pattern of cancer can be described in a number of ways:

- *Incidence* – the number of new cases in each year per head of the population or usually, to make comparisons easier, per 100,000 or per million heads.

- *Mortality* – the number of people who die of that cancer in each year per head of the population or per 100,000 people.

- *Prevalence* – the number of cancers that exist at any one time in a particular population, which will depend both on the incidence (new cases developing) and the mortality.

At first glance it might seem easy to produce this information. In fact it can be surprisingly difficult. Death certificates ought to provide accurate information about the mortality from cancer in a whole population when records are kept. In fact death-certificate information can be quite inaccurate and is not always collected well.

Many countries have developed a system of cancer registration in order to collect information about cancer incidence. The information is collected from hospital records, death certificates and hospital laboratories, and great attention is now given to cross-checking and comparing information to ensure its reliability. Most European countries collect information on mortality. However, even within Europe, we find differences in national commitment to collecting such data (Luxembourg, for example, does not have cancer registration). Perhaps the countries with the most outstanding record of accurate collection of valuable information are Denmark and Scotland. In England and Wales the regional cancer registries are broadly accurate, but some registries are better than others. Cancer registration is improving rapidly in the new southern European members of the European Community, such as Portugal and Greece.

In the United States national cancer registration began towards the end of the nineteenth century, but it was not until

1933 that information was collected in all states and only as late as 1979 was a national registry of all cancer deaths established.

Analytical Studies

In the performance of analytical studies epidemiologists move from the demanding chores of collecting accurate information into the realms of designing studies that seek to answer important individual questions about the causes of cancer. In this area they will usually have an idea to test – a hypothesis about some possible causative factor. The focus shifts from whole nations or whole regions to a much more closely defined group of individuals. By collecting a great deal more information about a rather smaller number of people (but not so small that our conclusions might be based on pure chance), it is possible not only to demonstrate links between particular factors and particular cancers but also to look carefully to see if there are any possible alternative links which have to be considered or excluded by careful work. A number of methods of performing analytical epidemiology are recognized and are worth mentioning to give the general flavour of this sort of work: cohort studies, case-control studies and intervention or experimental studies.

Cohort Studies

A group of people (usually hundreds or even thousands) are identified who have either been exposed to a particular risk factor or who may become exposed to some risk during the study. They are then followed up carefully and the development of the particular cancer or cancers under study is recorded and compared to that in a similar group of people who have not suffered any exposure to the relevant risk. Although this sounds like a simple operation, collecting together the information on an adequate number of people and following them up for a long enough period is difficult, laborious and expensive. These studies may look at groups of people who are known to have been exposed to a risk already – workers exposed to a chemical for instance. On the other hand, they may take a group of people in a job and then look at their exposure to a risk as it develops. Further follow-up then checks for cancer incidence. This second kind of study – called a *prospective cohort study* – can be particularly accurate.

Case-control Studies

In this method the group of people about whom information is collected are those who are already suffering from the particular cancer. They are then matched to another group of people who do not have the cancer but who are similar in other aspects such as age, sex and often social group. The group of patients with the cancer (the cases) are then compared to the group who do not have the cancer (the controls) in terms of their previous exposures to all sorts of factors. If the cases have had more exposure to a particular factor than the controls, it suggests that that particular factor is linked to the cancer. Again, it sounds easy but collecting the information is a laborious task and choosing controls is full of pitfalls. If the groups are not properly matched then misleading links can be suggested. A particular pitfall is choosing groups of people when they come to hospital. Hospital-based control groups may be very unrepresentative of the general population.

Intervention or Experimental Studies

These studies represent the most difficult but in many ways the most informative of all forms of analytic epidemiology.

Here, two very similar groups of people are identified, often by computer-generated methods, randomly allocating people into one or other of the groups. With the consent of the people involved, one half are asked to undertake a change in their lifestyle. Perhaps a particular dietary element may be changed for that group alone, on the theory that that dietary element may be related to cancer. The people are then studied for a long period of time to see if there is any difference in the medical outcomes between the two groups. Since the groups of people were essentially identical at the beginning, any differences that emerge are very likely to be linked directly to the change that was introduced for one group alone. This is precise science which can give accurate answers, but it is fraught with many human problems. The first of these is ethical. If there is a strong and genuine suspicion that the intervention may be helpful, and that only one group will benefit from it, many physicians would feel it morally wrong to perform such studies. Equally, if, as is essential in all medical research, the people involved are fully informed of the experiment being undertaken, many may feel unwilling to join. This means that accruing numbers of people into these studies may prove difficult. It is also extremely difficult to choose the right point in time at which to undertake an intervention study. If the risk factor being studied is very likely to be associated with cancer, then the ethical constraints will make it too difficult to perform the study, since no researcher will want just one group of people to benefit from an intervention study which leaves the other group exposed to a highly probable risk. If, on the other hand, the information about the risk factor is very preliminary and perhaps weak, then there may not be sufficient reason to deploy the resources required for an intervention study in order to evaluate it fully. In a few circumstances the right point has been identified and there are currently major debates about whether intervention studies to test a number of other important theories are appropriate.

Epidemiology: How Conclusive?

We have outlined the ways in which epidemiologists can describe and analyse the vast amount of information now being collected about human cancer in populations. Can they produce conclusions from these studies? The answer is: probably not from any single study. Only the intervention studies can generate precise answers to precise questions, and these are few and far between and very difficult to perform adequately. In most other situations, conclusions are reached by adding together the suggestions derived from the descriptive and the analytical studies, often when several such studies have been performed. In addition, facts that emerge from experimental science in the laboratory or from clinical sciences often need to be built into the overall equation before conclusions can be reached.

Why are single descriptive studies often fallible? Even if we find that one population or group is more prone to cancer than another, we may have considerable difficulty in determining which factor (or combination of factors) is responsible for the higher incidence of the disease. It is very unlikely that the two populations or groups will be different from each other in only one respect or in a very limited number of ways. The number of variations between them (both environmental and genetic) is likely to be enormous. The population which is more exposed to the risk (or combination of risks) in which the cancer epidemiologist is interested may be different from the other population in a host of other ways that could just as easily account for the higher incidence of cancer. A cancer may have many interacting causes, some of which are, as yet, unknown. The epidemiologist may thus overlook some of the variations between the exposure characteristics of the two populations which might explain the different rates of cancer.

The ideas that we have to test in epidemiology have to come either from initial observations in populations (like the connection between smoking and lung cancer, or between occupation and certain cancers) or from the laboratory. We often do not have precise enough ideas to test, and some of our ideas may be wrong. We are fortunate when a clinician comes up with a clue like that which occurred for Percival Pott from his observations of chimney-sweeps. Similar astute clinical observations have led on to other detailed epidemiological studies which have reached helpful conclusions. The link between bone cancer and the use of radioactive substances in manufacturing was first described this way, as was the link between asbestos and the very serious form of chest cancer known as mesothelioma.

The central difficulty in interpreting the results of epidemiological studies lies in distinguishing whether a link that appears to exist between a risk factor and a cancer is truly a causal one. For everybody except epidemiologists, this problem requires quite a lot of explanation. The studies may show that a particular group within the population is more likely to get a particular kind of cancer. Let us say, for example, that the members of a particular occupation are more likely to get stomach cancer. Some particular feature of that occupation attracts attention. Let us suppose that the occupation is associated with extensive foreign travel. We know that the members of that occupation are more likely to have stomach cancer than the general population, so we might look for a link between the number of miles flown in an aeroplane and the incidence of stomach cancer. We will find that there is an association. These people travel abroad much more than people whose jobs keep them at home. Does air travel cause stomach cancer? The link is there from this epidemiological study but it may not mean that air travel causes cancer. There may be something else about this population which explains that high incidence of stomach cancer. Could it be that their foreign travel takes them to parts of the world where the diet is very unusual?

Perhaps they are eating something abroad which is associated with stomach cancer. Perhaps, on the other hand, these high-flying foreign travellers are very well paid and are therefore living lavish lifestyles, eating lots of rich food and drinking lots of alcohol. Is it this that is the causative factor for their stomach cancer? The point we are making is simply that the establishment of a link between a cancer and a particular feature of someone's life can never prove in itself that that link is responsible. If the link is a very strong one and if it seems to be sensible in biological terms (perhaps diet is more likely than air travel to be a factor in stomach cancer), then it can be an important clue, but it doesn't demonstrate proof of the cause, and much more work is necessary before we can assert with confidence that there is a causative link.

We should emphasize that we have used the example of air travel and stomach cancer simply as an illustration of the need to be careful in interpreting epidemiological evidence. There is no need for members of the travel industry to go rushing off to see their doctors!

Some of the problems which we encounter in trying to prove causal links loom very large at the present time. The best example is the possible link between dietary fat and breast cancer. We will discuss this topic in detail in a later chapter but one point can be made here. Breast cancer is much commoner in countries where women eat a lot of animal fat. This might mean that animal fat causes breast cancer. However, the countries in which we eat a lot of animal fat are also the wealthy countries of the world and they have many other distinctive features. Work patterns are different and leisure activities are different. In wealthy countries women are much more likely to own a television set. It follows therefore that those countries where television ownership is high have a high incidence of breast cancer. Television doesn't cause breast cancer. The link exists because of the association with high standards of living. A high intake of animal fat may or may not turn out to be a cause of breast cancer; unravelling this factor from other factors which might contribute to the development of breast cancer is a major target of epidemiological studies at present.

THE GEOGRAPHY OF CANCER

We have already mentioned that there are huge variations between different countries and different communities. In this section we are going to gather together some statistics and those who have no wish to try to digest or, worse still, remember large collections of numbers, are encouraged to move swiftly on to the next chapter. However, no book on the cancer problem can be complete without at least giving an idea about the distribution of cancers in different countries and the types of cancers which constitute the main problems.

The European Community

The 'Europe against Cancer' programme was launched in 1987 as a major effort to control cancer in the EC. Prevention was the target, and tobacco, alcohol, diet, occupation and screening were the factors of greatest interest. As a baseline for this effort workers from the Danish Institute of Cancer Epidemiology and the International Agency for Research on Cancer in Lyon prepared a report, 'Cancer in the European Community and its Member States'.* With the permission of these authors we will quote here extensively from their report. Many of their conclusions were based on estimates, because not all EC coun-

---

* Jensen, O.M., Estève, J., Moller, H., and Renard, H. (1990), 'Cancer in the European Community and its member states', *European Journal of Cancer*, 26: 1167–256.

tries collect precise information on cancer incidence. None the less, they concluded that the study 'leaves little doubt that cancer represents a major health problem in the EC and its member states. The burden of cancer on society, measured by the number of new cases arising every year may be some 20 per cent higher than hitherto assumed.'

In the current twelve-member European Community, there were 750,000 deaths from cancer in 1980 and an estimated 1,200,000 new cases of cancer. Statistical methods can be employed to make allowance for the differing ages of the populations in the different countries and, when this is done, a rank order of cancer incidence and cancer deaths in men and women can be prepared; we have shown this in Figure 6.

It emerges that the risk of dying from cancer in the European Community among men is highest in Luxembourg, Belgium, France and the Netherlands and lowest in Portugal, Greece, Spain and Ireland. The difference is quite large and the incidence of cancer is 55 per cent higher among the French than among the Portuguese. The risk of dying from cancer is 40 per cent lower in women than in men in the European Community and the highest incidence rates in women are seen in Luxembourg, the UK, Denmark and Ireland, while the lowest are seen in Spain, Greece and Portugal. There are striking disparities between countries in the differences in cancer incidence between sexes. French men are twice as likely to get cancer as French women while in Denmark men and women have a very similar incidence.

Among men, the commonest cancer is in the lung, followed by cancer in the prostate, colon and bladder. Among women, the leading site is in the breast, followed by cancer of the colon, cancer in the stomach and gynaecological cancers. This pattern in broad terms is similar for different countries but there are important differences. Lung cancer is the commonest cancer in men in every state and breast cancer is the commonest

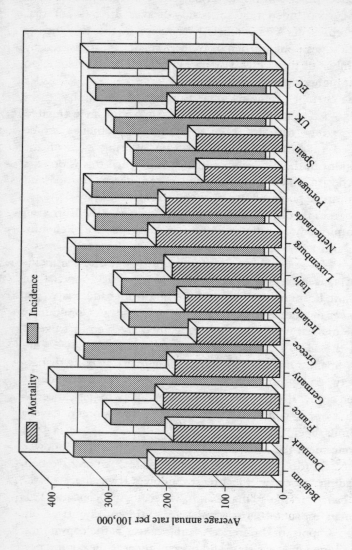

Figure 6 (a) Estimated incidence and mortality for all cancer except skin cancer in men.

(From Jensen *et al.*, 'Cancer in the European Community and its member states', *European Journal of Cancer*, 1990.)

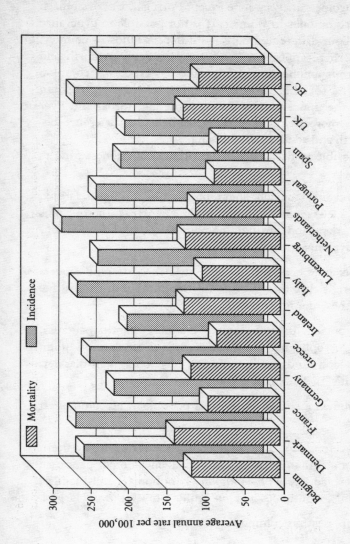

Figure 6 (b) Estimated incidence and mortality for all cancer except skin cancer in women.

(From Jensen *et al.*, 'Cancer in the European Community and its member states', *European Journal of Cancer*, 1990.)

cancer in women in every state except Portugal, where stomach cancer is commoner in women. It is not possible to generalize entirely about differences between different kinds of country. However, there appears to be a contrast between north and south Europe among men. Lung cancer is especially common in the north, together with rectal cancer, whereas in the south cancer of the upper part of the intestine and throat and liver cancer are more frequent. Among women, the difference between north and south is less striking.

It is possible to list in order the twenty commonest cancers in men:

lung, prostate, stomach, colon, bladder, liver, mouth, larynx, rectum, leukaemia, kidney, brain, pancreas, oesophagus (gullet), non-Hodgkin lymphoma, testis, melanoma, Hodgkin's, myeloma and gall-bladder.

It is important, however, to note that the different cancers have different cure rates so that for the number of deaths due to cancer the order is different:

lung, stomach, prostate, colon, bladder, mouth, pancreas, rectum, oesophagus (gullet), leukaemia, liver, larynx, brain, kidney, non-Hodgkin lymphoma, myeloma, gall-bladder, Hodgkin's, melanoma and testis.

Among women a similar exercise is possible. The commonest cancers are:

breast, colon, stomach, ovary, cervix uteri, corpus uteri, liver, lung, brain, rectum, leukaemia, melanoma, pancreas, kidney, bladder, non-Hodgkin lymphoma, gall-bladder, Hodgkin's, mouth, oesophagus (gullet), myeloma and larynx.

For women, death is commonest from cancers in:

breast, colon, lung, stomach, ovary, cervix uteri, pancreas, leukaemia, rectum, brain, liver, corpus uteri, gall bladder, kidney, non-Hodgkin lymphoma, bladder, oesophagus (gullet), myeloma, mouth, melanoma, Hodgkin's and larynx.

Comparing different cancers between European countries can be linked to probable causes. Liver cancer is a good example: it is common in Greece, France, Italy and Spain, possibly because of a high intake of wine in these countries. This link is probably a real and causal one, and we shall be discussing it later. Nevertheless, this link probably doesn't explain all the differences. There are other cancers associated with alcohol, including mouth cancers, and these are not particularly common in Greece. It may be that chronic liver infection with hepatitis viruses is a factor in some countries. Looking at cancer of the larynx a similar message emerges, with the French, Spanish, Italian and now Portuguese men having an alarmingly high incidence of this cancer, which is otherwise not one of the most frequent in other countries. The risk factors here are probably both tobacco and alcohol, which seem to interact to make the risk of cancer of the larynx especially high for the French.

Bad news comes for the northern Europeans when we look at lung cancer. This most frequent of cancers in men is particularly common in the United Kingdom and the Low Countries. In these high-risk countries the International Agency for Research on Cancer estimates that some 85 per cent of the cases are due to cigarette smoking.

Melanoma of the skin in Europe presents us with an interesting paradox. The high-risk countries are in northern Europe, particularly Scandinavia, the Netherlands, Germany and the UK. We shall see later that melanoma of the skin develops as a result of excessive exposure to sunlight; yet people living in the sunny climates in southern Europe appear to have a low incidence. The explanation lies in differences between the type of complexion found in the north and the south. The people who get melanoma appear to be those with light complexions who have intermittent exposures, leading to sunburn in young individuals and a tendency to freckle and to burn rather than tan. In North America and Australia, where the racial mix is more evenly spread through the country, the incidence of melanoma gets higher as the equator is approached and the sun gets stronger. The opposite is seen in Europe because the northern Europeans have light complexions and for them occasional exposure, perhaps on holiday in southern Europe, appears to be most harmful.

The European picture is therefore one of variation which can be quite large and which is often explained by readily identifiable factors which affect the communities, perhaps particularly alcohol, cigarettes and exposure of fair skin to sunlight. Since many of these are easily identified and avoidable we may already be part of the way down our road towards identifying the preventable causes of cancer.

Intercontinental Variations

The list of contrasts that can be drawn when the variation in national incidence of cancers is examined across the whole world is endless. We have looked in detail at Europe and in this section we will give a few examples to illustrate that intercontinental differences can be even more dramatic than international differences.

The International Agency for Research on Cancer regularly publishes a compendium of cancer incidence in five continents, the most recent edition of which was in 1987. From these published figures it is possible to pull out some striking examples between the highest incidence and the lowest incidence across the world. The most dramatic is malignant melanoma, for which the lowest known incidence is in Japan (2 cases in every 1,000,000 people every year) and the highest known incidence is in Queensland (309 cases in every 1,000,000 people every year); the difference is 150-fold. This is attributable, at least in part, to the combination of light-skinned people exposed to very bright sunshine in Queensland near the equator compared with darker-complexioned people living in the less sunny climes of Japan. Cancers arising in the back of the nasal cavity are common in Hong Kong (300 in every 1,000,000 people every year) but rare in the UK (3 in every 1,000,000 each year). The explanation for this difference is not so simple but may relate to chronic virus infection with a virus known as the Epstein–Barr virus, and may not exclude other factors such as dietary factors and genetic factors. The Chinese are not always on the wrong side of the equation. For instance, with cancer of the prostate gland in men 900 US blacks out of every 1,000,000 develop the disease each year but 13 in every 1,000,000 Chinese. We find the world's highest incidence of stomach cancer in Japan (820 per 1,000,000 per year). This is to be compared with a much lower incidence elsewhere, particularly in the Middle East (3–4 per 1,000,000 per year).

The range for the common cancers can also be very large. The highest incidence of lung cancer is 1,100 per 1,000,000 per year in the US but only 58 per 1,000,000 per year in India; similarly colon cancer is 340 per 1,000,000 per year in the US and only 18 per 1,000,000 per year in India; breast cancer is 900 per 1,000,000 women per year in Hawaii but only 14 per 1,000,000 per year in parts of the Middle East. Where we are able to pin down the causes of these variations, the potential for prevention is obvious and large. Where the causes are unknown, the room for research is equally large and potentially equally rewarding.

United Kingdom

The distribution of cancers within individual countries can be very striking. Sometimes these distributions can attract a great deal of publicity. Perhaps the best known example in the United Kingdom is the relationship of childhood leukaemia, which is reported to be unusually high in the vicinity of nuclear power stations: the occurrence of childhood leukaemia around the nuclear processing plant at Sellafield has been reported to be as much as ten times the national average, whereas in the neighbourhood of other nuclear installations the incidence is about 20 per cent above the national average. The explanation for this is still not clear. The association with parental employment in the nuclear installations has been the cause of much discussion but is not yet settled. The arguments are usually based on very small numbers of cases which makes it difficult to draw firm conclusions.

Very detailed studies of the distribution of leukaemias and lymphomas in England and Wales have been carried out by the Leukaemia Research Fund Centre for Clinical Epidemiology run by our colleagues Ray Cartwright and Freda Alexander. One of the most striking features of their analysis is that many of these conditions have a relatively high incidence rate in the county of Somerset. The explanation for this is not forthcoming, but they have studied it in great detail and it appears that the high rates are real and call for further study to see if explanations can be found. It should be emphasized that these are relatively uncommon diseases and that while the higher incidence rates in Somerset are a source of concern and justify very detailed further work, in absolute terms the number of people affected is quite small and should not be a cause for general alarm in that part of the world.

What about commoner cancers? Lung cancer is the commonest cancer in men and careful studies of its geographic distribution in the United Kingdom have been performed for many years. The map (Figure 7) is taken from a paper written by Dr Tony Swerdlow in the *British Journal of Cancer* in 1991 and shows the relative frequency of lung cancer in young men in

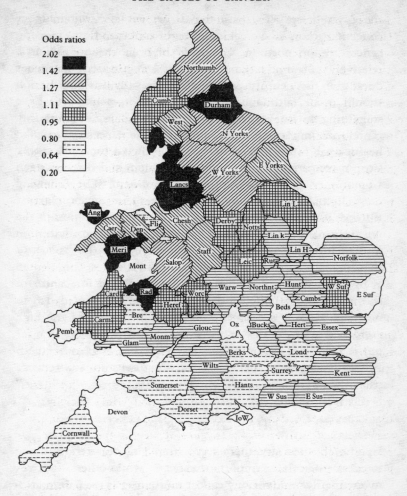

Figure 7 Map of the risk of lung cancer in men aged under forty-five years in England and Wales, 1968–81, by county of residence.

(From Swerdlow *et al.*, 'Geographic distribution of lung and stomach cancers in England and Wales over 50 years: changing and unchanging patterns', *British Journal of Cancer*, 1991.)

the 1970s and 1980s, with the darker spots showing higher concentrations. The strikingly high concentrations of lung cancer in the north of England are obvious and this is a relatively new finding, having been less apparent in earlier decades in this century. We do not know why this distribution should occur, although we believe that it is likely to have something to do with the pattern of smoking. It certainly represents important information for those seeking to plan health care. Similar maps can be constructed for most cancer sites in countries like the United Kingdom and the European Community where accurate records are kept. The following map (Figure 8) shows the distribution of lung cancer across Europe, which again brings out the high concentration in the northern part of England but shows further the concentration in Scotland and in northern European countries. For cancer of the breast in women the high concentration in the United Kingdom in general is apparent (Figure 9) and for cancer of the oesophagus (gullet) in men the very high incidence in northern France is clear (Figure 10). The causes of the high incidence of cancer of the breast in the UK are not at all clear but the cause of cancer of the oesophagus in men in northern France is very likely to be associated with alcohol and tobacco use.

CHANGE OVER TIME

During this century there have been striking trends in the incidence of certain important cancers, while others have remained fairly steady. Lung cancer mortality has risen dramatically in the last fifty to sixty years. Colorectal cancer (cancer of the large intestine and rectum) increased in most of the Western world in the 1930s and 1940s but has been steady for the last thirty years. There seems to have been an increase in cancer of the prostate gland in men between 1930 and 1950 but this may

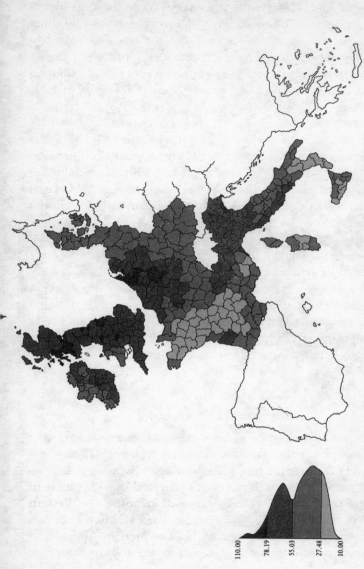

Figure 8 Map of mortality from cancer of the lung in men.

(Reproduced with permission from Muir *et al.*, *Atlas of Cancer Mortality in the European Economic Community*, International Agency for Research on Cancer, Scientific Publications No. 107, 1992.

110.00
78.19
55.03
27.48
10.00

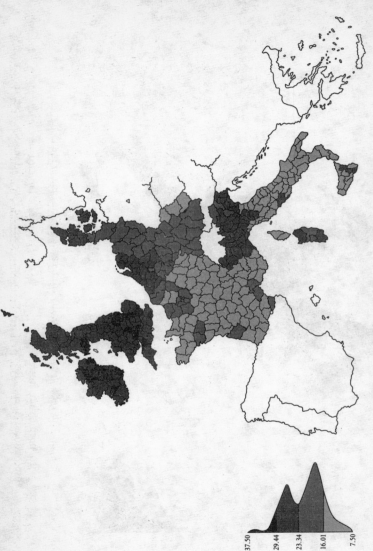

Figure 9 Map of mortality from cancer of the breast in women.

(Reproduced with permission from Muir *et al.*, *Atlas of Cancer Mortality in the European Economic Community*, International Agency for Research on Cancer, Scientific Publications No. 107, 1992.

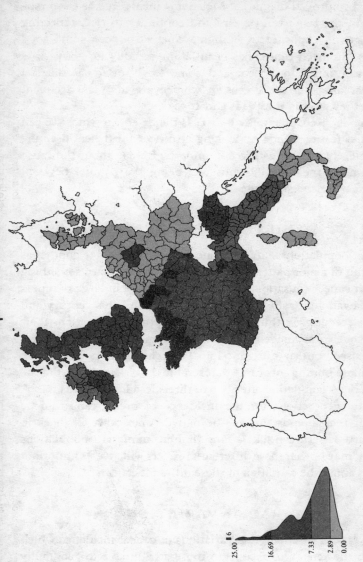

Figure 10 Map of mortality from cancer of the oesophagus (gullet) in men.

(Reproduced with permission from Muir *et al.*, *Atlas of Cancer Mortality in the European Economic Community*, International Agency for Research on Cancer, Scientific Publications No. 107, 1992.

reflect improved diagnosis. Melanoma incidence has risen rapidly in the last twenty years and continues to rise, reflecting changes in exposure to sunlight. There has been some good news. Stomach cancer has been falling steadily for sixty years and continues to do so, and some kinds of gynaecological cancer affecting the uterus in women are now less frequent than they were in the 1940s and 1950s.

In a later chapter we will discuss the extent to which we can predict future trends by looking at cancer incidence in young people. These trends provide important clues about the cause of cancer, the most obvious one being the parallel between lung cancer and smoking.

SHIFTING POPULATIONS

When populations shift from one part of the world to another as a result of major patterns of emigration we may learn something about cancer causation. The Japanese moved in large numbers to Hawaii and California in the early part of this century and again recently. Within a few decades of these emigrations their previously low incidence of bowel cancers and of breast cancers increased, but at different rates. Large bowel cancer in the Japanese immigrants came to resemble the risk in the rest of the American population after two to three decades, whereas it took several generations for the incidence of breast cancer to be about the same as that of the native Americans. Changes in dietary pattern can take a long time in immigrant populations and it may be that these differential effects will give us important clues about the causation of these different cancers.

RACIAL VARIATION

The task of disentangling variations in cancer incidence which might be related to race from those attributable to geography is always going to present problems if each race stays in its country of origin. The best opportunity comes from the United States with its great mix of different immigrant races. The figures for the United States have been examined in detail by American epidemiologists and some startling variations have been found. These may of course still not be attributable purely to the racial differences but could reflect the cultural, dietary and economic differences between the different groups within the country. Having acknowledged that we must be cautious in interpreting the causes of the variations, we find that, in general, American blacks have a much higher cancer incidence (5,000 per 1,000,000 per year) than American Indians who represent the other extreme (2,000 per 1,000,000 per year). The overall descending order of cancer incidence among American races goes blacks, whites, Hawaiians, Japanese, Chinese, Hispanics, Filipinos and American Indians. However, this pattern is not uniform across all cancer sites, and for cancer of the stomach, for instance, the Japanese, Hawaiians and American Indians represent the highest-risk group while the whites are at lower risk. For melanoma of the skin, the white-skinned races are, as expected, most vulnerable, whereas blacks have a very low incidence indeed, as do most of the other races with more pigmented skins.

THE SOCIOLOGY OF CANCER

Wealth will determine environment both between countries and within countries; again, nowhere is the effect of wealth more apparent than in the United States. As ever, it is difficult to separate this factor from those of race or occupation.

The sociology of cancer has been the subject of intense research in the United States, where the risk of getting cancer was studied in relation to socio-economic status in the *Third National Cancer Survey* (published in the early 1970s). Irrespective of age or geographical location, a higher cancer incidence was observed in people with low income, with a steady fall in incidence as income increased, and with the lowest incidence of all being found in those with high incomes. The difference was about 20 per cent between the lowest and the highest income groups but was not uniform between different cancer sites. In men, the low-income groups did particularly badly for cancer of the lung, stomach and oesophagus, probably reflecting more smoking and drinking in the lower-income groups. In women, cancer of the cervix was more frequent in lower-income groups but there were two important exceptions to the general trend, with cancer of the breast and cancer of the body of uterus being less frequent in the low-income groups (perhaps reflecting nutritional differences or differences in child-bearing and menstruation). We will say more about this in later chapters.

THE IDENTIFIABLE CAUSES OF CANCER

The question the reader will ask at this point is 'Given all this epidemiological study, do we know the causes of cancer?' Broadly the answer is 'yes' in many circumstances and for many cancers, and the opportunities for prevention that this understanding generates are there to be taken. We do not always know how the factors that have been identified by the epidemiological studies discussed in this chapter link up to what is being learned in the laboratories of the molecular biologists. This connection is being made rapidly and will be increasingly clear by the end of the century. Epidemiology has been very successful in discovering or confirming which features of our lives in the Western world can be now identified as causes of cancer. Many of these will be looked at in subsequent chapters but a summary here will serve as an introduction for some readers and will perhaps be sufficient for others.

Tobacco

Tobacco smoking has been shown to be the cause of most lung cancers in the Western world, particularly in men, but the link is becoming increasingly apparent in the developing countries. Probably 40 per cent of all cancer deaths in men and some 20 per cent in women are attributable to smoking, with the majority being caused by lung cancer, but with important and well-demonstrated links to cancers of the larynx, mouth, gullet and bladder, and with some suggestion also that there is a link to cancers of the kidney, cervix, nose and even the stomach. Tobacco sniffing and chewing also cause cancer, and smokers can quite possibly cause cancers in those who live with them by the process of passive smoke inhalation. Constituents of tobacco smoke can be found in the body fluids of non-smokers.

We will make clear recommendations about tobacco for those interested in avoiding cancer risks. (See p.76 ff.)

Diet

Experimental studies undertaken in a number of countries suggest that dietary alteration can alter the growth of tumours, and links between a Western diet and some cancers have become apparent. However, it is not proving quite so easy to demonstrate precise links between specific elements of a diet and specific cancers. Dietary fat may be a factor in breast and bowel cancer but there may also be other explanations for some of the links between these cancers and our way of life in the Western world. Cooked-meat intake may be a factor in bowel cancer and fibre or starch may be protective against this cancer. Obesity is a risk factor for some cancers in women, particularly cancer of the body of the uterus. Whether being overweight causes cancer by altering circulating hormones is not yet clear. Green vegetables and fresh fruit seem to be associated with a lower incidence of several cancers but the link is a complicated one. Vitamins and minerals in diet are also being studied but we cannot claim to have all the answers as to how they may prevent the development of cancer.

Our recommendations about diet and nutrition will be cautious.

Hormones

A few hormones can certainly cause cancer. When large quantities of the female hormone oestrogen were given for medical reasons during pregnancy, rare kinds of cancer were later found in the daughters of these women. Large quantities of oestrogens which were formerly given to women for menopausal symptoms undoubtedly caused cancer in the uterus although newer preparations do not. Oral contraceptives represent a complicated case, perhaps involving a real increased risk of breast cancer, particularly in young people. On the other hand, the Pill is capable of reducing the risk of ovarian cancer and cancer of the body of the uterus. Both risks and benefits can therefore be claimed for the Pill and controversy about its use is likely to continue.

At a more subtle level, it is possible that some of the effects of child-bearing may include a reduction in some cancer risks, probably generated by changing hormone levels. This is particularly apparent in cancer of the ovary, where having been pregnant appears to be protective.

Sex

Sexual activity has been extensively investigated as a factor in the cause of certain cancers, particularly cancer of the neck of uterus. Certainly, the number of sexual partners appears to be an association. In a woman with only a single lifelong sexual partner, the number of partners that her one sexual partner has had also seems to affect her risk. How this leads to a cancer, and particularly whether the cancer is caused by transfer of a virus, is the subject of current research focusing particularly on the human papilloma virus. The transfer of infectious agents which give rise to AIDS must also be considered under this heading because people with AIDS can get unusual types of cancer.

Radiation

The effects of radiation as a cause of cancer are probably as well understood as anything else, except perhaps those of smoking. Survivors of the atomic bombs and people given low doses of radiation for medical treatments decades ago all have a higher chance of getting certain cancers, particularly leukaemias. Ordinary diagnostic X-rays now deliver only tiny amounts of radiation and appear not to have any adverse effect in adults but it is wise to keep them to the minimum necessary. Uranium miners seem to get more lung cancer than would be expected and there is currently much research, which is not yet conclusive, into a connection between cancer and the indoor levels of some radioactive gases (such as radon) rising from rocks. One of the difficulties in dealing with radiation as a cause of cancer is uncertainty about the relationship between the dose of radiation received and the level of increased cancer risk. Under some circumstances, very low doses may be associated with subtle effects on cancer risk.

Protection against radiation is well established in the workplace but more research work is needed on the effects of low levels of radiation. The protection of society as a whole against the possible hazards of radiation obviously raises complex economic, political and social issues.

Sunlight

Ultraviolet irradiation from the sun is the main cause of skin cancers, including melanoma. Just how certain we can be about this and how we can avoid its effects will be discussed in Chapter 6. Some fairly significant recommendations can now be made.

Alcohol

Alcohol contributes to cancers of the upper digestive tract, particularly in combination with smoking. It probably also contributes to cancers of the liver, mainly, but perhaps not exclusively, through causing cirrhosis of the liver. There is little doubt that advice on the avoidance of heavy drinking is sound if we wish to reduce cancer risk as well as the other risks with which drinking is associated.

Occupations

Cancer epidemiology really began with Percival Pott and his chimney-sweeps, and, for many researchers, creating a safe workplace and eliminating risks is a central purpose of epidemiological studies. Chemical dyes and asbestos have been identified as causes of cancer and eliminated in the workplace, but constant vigilance is still in order. New and stringent regulations permitting only limited exposure to substances hazardous to health are now in force in many Western European countries, and their extension to Eastern Europe represents a significant financial, political and medical challenge.

Environmental Pollution

Most of the factors that are hazardous in the workplace are found in lower concentrations in the general environment and may well contribute to cancer risk. Atmospheric pollution probably plays only a limited role in lung cancer, but asbestos in the general environment has undoubtedly contributed to the level of risk.

Infections

Simple infections do not cause cancer. Pneumonias and urinary infections, for instance, are usually caused by bacteria and there is no evidence that such infections predispose to cancer in any way. Animal cancers can be caused by viruses but, as we indicated in Chapter 2, human cancers are not usually caused by viruses. There are, however, some notable exceptions to this general statement. The virus described by Epstein and Barr (Epstein–Barr virus, EBV) probably causes a rare cancer of the lymph glands, particularly in Africa, and may cause cancer of the nasal passages among the Chinese. Hepatitis B virus infection, when chronic, probably contributes to the high incidence of liver cancers in the Far East, the evidence for this being a most convincing cohort study in Taiwan. Rare types of leukaemia, particularly in Japan and the Caribbean, have been linked to infection with a particular kind of virus (human T lymphotrophic virus type 1), which seems to be spread early in life but which may also, like AIDS, be spread by sexual activity and drug abuse. AIDS infection predisposes patients to a number of cancers of a rare kind which may be very difficult indeed to treat. As indicated above, viruses are being investigated as a possible explanation for a link between cancer of the neck of the womb and multiple sexual partners. It should be emphasized that human cancer is not in any simple way an infectious disease, that patients with cancer do not require isolation and that people need not be concerned about sharing homes or workplaces with cancer patients.

Drugs

Very few medicines have been implicated as causing cancers but there are three groups of drugs where cancer is probably an important and often unavoidable side effect. Hormones have already been mentioned. The very drugs that are used for treating cancers by chemotherapy include some (particularly those known as alkylating agents) which interfere with DNA and, hence, with some genes. Cases of leukaemia and other cancers are being discovered as a delayed after-effect of such drugs in patients who have been cured of their first cancer by such chemotherapy. Not all the drugs used in chemotherapy have this effect and modern treatments appear to have reduced the risks considerably. The third group which may put people at risk are those drugs which are used to suppress the body's immune function. These are used for patients who have had transplants and in such patients, particularly those with kidney transplants, certain rare kinds of cancer, including those known as lymphoma, have been found. As a result of the risks, these patients have to be monitored very carefully.

Genetic Susceptibility

Most cancers are not inherited. Environmental influences are far more important. However, we must consider genetics in relation to cancer in three ways. First, we have already mentioned that when cells within the body undergo malignant change and then divide to form two daughter cells, these daughter cells will retain the genetic features of the parent cells. In this sense cancer is a genetic disease between the cells. When we use the term 'daughter' in this context, this is simply scientific jargon for cells within one person. We are not implying that parents pass on genetic risks to daughters.

The second role of genetics lies in the genetic make-up of

the person at risk. It may be the case that the genetic make-up of individuals makes them more or less susceptible to cancer-causing agents in the environment. A good example is that of skin cancer. Some individuals and races inherit dark pigmentation which is capable of preventing the cancer-causing effects of ultraviolet sunlight. Black people very rarely get the kind of skin cancer called melanoma. Other races are born with complexions which mean they are at risk from the effects of environmental cancer-causing agents. Fair-skinned people are at risk from melanoma if they get sunburn. This is the second sense in which we can consider cancer in relation to genes.

Finally, we turn now to those cancers which are truly inherited by being passed from parents to their children. There are over two hundred disorders which have been linked to cancer and have been shown to be inherited by a single gene being passed between parents and their children. However, they are all extremely rare. They will nevertheless have a dramatic and devastating impact on the unfortunate families in which the genes occur and such families require detailed medical attention and support.

Many Diseases/Many Causes

In Chapter 2, we described how cancers evolve in several stages as a result of changes in their molecular biology. These changes are usually brought about by several causes. These may be 'positive' causes like the presence of chemicals in cigarette smoke or 'negative' causes like the absence of fibre from the diet. The different causes will interact with each other and the outcome may also be affected by the genetic make-up of the individual.

The impression we want to leave is one of cancer as many different diseases, each with different causes and, in most cases, several different causes which will interact to produce the cancer and to influence how it behaves once established.

*

We hope by now to have given our readers the impression that a great deal is known about the causes of cancer, both in the laboratory and as a result of studies of the occurrence of cancer in the populations of the world. Important causes have been identified and are open to preventive measures. We do not know all the answers, and the methods of study that are available to us are highly demanding. Great efforts are being made in the laboratory, in hospitals and in epidemiology centres and cancer registries around the world to define the causes of cancer as precisely as possible. Steady success is being achieved.

In subsequent chapters we shall try to show in more detail how strong or weak is the evidence in each area, and will base our advice on the strength of the evidence.

4
Smoking and Cancer

Lung cancer has been one of the most important epidemics of the twentieth century. Late-nineteenth-century physicians and surgeons rarely diagnosed lung cancer and, even though techniques for making the alternative and more frequent diagnosis of tuberculosis were only partly developed at that time, it is unlikely that they were failing to make the diagnosis and much more likely that lung cancer was a medical rarity at that time. Now lung cancer is, in all probability, the commonest cancer in the world, with nearly 700,000 cases per year. In the United Kingdom, it accounts for 25 per cent of cancer deaths.

The epidemic has been especially damaging. The disease strikes down men who are still economically productive and have dependent families. Sadly, the outlook for a patient diagnosed as having lung cancer remains one of the most dismal of all cancer diagnoses. Whereas the surgeon may hope to cure a third or a half of all of the patients whom he treats for other common cancers, the situation is quite different with lung cancer. When the diagnosis is made, no more than one quarter of patients have a disease that can be removed by surgery. Even when surgery is carried out and it seems that the cancer has been removed, only about one quarter of those patients are cured. Overall, less than 10 per cent of patients will be cured by surgery.

Other means of treating lung cancer have been equally unsuccessful. Radiotherapy has been applied vigorously in a wide range of doses and with a wide range of schedules for the last fifty years. Although the treatments have become simpler and safer, and in many ways more sophisticated, very few patients are cured by radiotherapy alone. The introduction of drugs for the treatment of lung cancer in the 1960s gave rise to great hope for the group of patients with a sub-group of very dangerous cancers known as small-cell lung cancers. Combinations of drugs have proved capable of producing frequent remissions for this group of lung cancer patients. The disease shrinks readily away when the drugs are used and, during the 1970s and 1980s, intensive research was directed to using this effect and trying to turn it into lasting remissions and cures. Such efforts have, however, been met with disappointment. Patients with small-cell lung cancer can usually expect remissions as a result of these combination chemotherapies, but very few are cured.

The scale of the epidemic of lung cancer is illustrated in Figure 11. The disease started to increase in the 1920s and 1930s and achieved its present epidemic proportions during the 1950s and 1960s. The number of deaths due to lung cancer is, however, beginning to show signs of a significant reduction. The graph shows the death rate against the number of cigarettes consumed; we must now accept that this indicates the clearest and most important explanation of this century's lung cancer epidemic.

There is an indisputable and strong link between lung cancer and smoking. In fact, almost all lung cancers are attributable to smoking and, if the smoking habit were dropped, lung cancer would revert to its former status as an infrequent diagnosis, of concern only to the individual patient and doctor. Instead, it remains one of the most overwhelming public-health issues facing the world as it moves towards the twenty-first century.

SMOKING AND LUNG CANCER

The Tobacco Connection Revealed

At the end of the Second World War the link between smoking and lung cancer was not widely recognized. The rapid increase in the frequency of lung cancer was a cause of some concern but doctors were among the heaviest smokers, and smoking as a cause was, oddly enough, overlooked. How the connection was made has been recently summarized by Sir Richard Doll, who was closely involved and the following account is based largely on his report.*

Tobacco had been in use for over three hundred years, but it was probably the advent of cigarettes at the beginning of the twentieth century that started the lung cancer epidemic. Perhaps the clearest warning had been sounded by a researcher named Pearl from Johns Hopkin's University in the United States in a scientific paper in 1938 in which he reported that, 'the smoking of tobacco was statistically associated with an impairment of life duration and the amount and degree of the impairment increased as the habitual amount of smoking increased'. Before the war, therefore, Pearl had told us that smoking shortened life and that the more we did it the more it was likely to do so, but nobody took much notice.

The change in attitudes can be dated to 1950 when five reports of the tobacco–cancer link were made and Sir Richard Doll and Sir Austen Bradford Hill concluded that smoking caused lung cancer. There was a change in approach to examining the relationship; and large studies, drawing on all the skills of epidemiologists, were established to follow large numbers of individuals over several years. By 1954 it was very clear that smoking caused lung cancer. Doctors played a part here in two

---

* Doll, R., *et al.*, 'Tobacco-related diseases', *Journal of Smoking-related Diseases*, 1991, 3–13.

ways. Doll and Hill were the investigators but one important group of subjects consisted of doctors. When it looked likely that smoking caused lung cancer, many doctors stopped quickly. Showing that this group then became less likely to get cancer than those who continued to smoke was a strong piece of evidence.

From that time on links between smoking and other diseases, including heart attacks and other cancers, were increasingly demonstrated, and the complex interaction between the three thousand different chemicals to be found in tobacco smoke and the dozens of illnesses with which tobacco is now associated began to unfold.

How Do We Know Smoking Causes Lung Cancer?

Unravelling the link between smoking and lung cancer has been one of the most successful exercises in the science of epidemiology. The part played by British scientific workers, most notably Sir Richard Doll from the University of Oxford, has been one of the most substantial contributions of British science to medicine. In Chapter 3 we set out to explain how epidemiologists can attribute a cause to a disease; the studies of smoking are a particularly compelling example of how this can be done.

- *Through this century the upward trend in lung cancer has followed the upward trend in smoking closely.*

- *The incidence of lung cancer is higher in smokers.* A large number of studies in analytical epidemiology all point in the same direction.

- *The more you smoke the more likely you are to get lung cancer.* This is true for the duration of smoking and the number of cigarettes smoked. The exact relationship between the

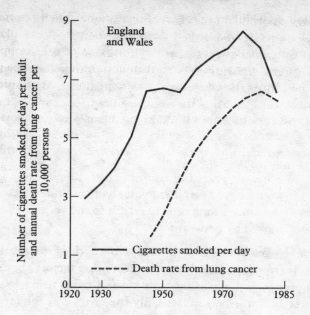

Figure 11 Smoking and lung cancer.

(From Doll, R., 'The prevention of cancer: opportunities and challenges', in Heller, T., Davey, B., and Bailey, L., eds., *Reducing the Risk of Cancers*, Hodder & Stoughton, 1989.)

number of cigarettes smoked and the increased risk of lung cancer can still be debated. People have smoked in different ways in different countries and discarded different amounts of the cigarettes. The tar content of cigarettes varies greatly and has fallen steadily in cigarettes smoked in Western Europe and the United States.

A recent estimate from the United States (report of the Surgeon General, 1989) says that regular cigarette smokers have more than a twenty times greater chance of getting lung cancer than lifelong non-smokers. The relationship between the number of cigarettes smoked and the risk is not a simple straight line. We cannot be precise about the relationship but Sir Richard Doll and his colleagues suggest that the likelihood of getting cancer from cigarette smoking rises according to a more complicated mathematical relationship known as a quadratic. Broadly this will mean that increasing the number of cigarettes smoked may have a disproportionate effect on the chance of getting lung cancer.

- *When you stop smoking your chance of getting lung cancer falls*. Within ten years the risk has fallen dramatically from what it would have been if smoking had continued although it may take quite a long time to return to the very small level of risk enjoyed by non-smokers.

- *Smoking low-tar cigarettes reduces the risk of lung cancer*. This is strong evidence because most other factors about the two groups – those using high-tar and those using low-tar cigarettes – will be similar. Only the change in the level of tar in cigarettes is likely to explain the change in lung cancer incidence which in low-tar smokers is reduced to about 60 per cent of the risk for patients smoking high-tar cigarettes.

- *Chemicals in cigarette tar are mutagenic and carcinogenic*. By this we mean that such chemicals alter genes and have been shown in the laboratory to produce cancer.

Lung Cancer in Non-smokers

People who do not smoke can get lung cancer, and careful observations involving large numbers of people in several countries suggest that the risk in non-smokers is of the order of 10–15 in every 100,000 people per year. Factors other than smoking are therefore obviously implicated. However, since the number of lung cancers in the Western population as a whole is about 100 per 100,000 per year, the impact of smoking is very great. If the number of cases expected in the population is calculated, a recent figure suggests that smoking is responsible for 93 per cent of lung cancers in men in the United Kingdom and 86 per cent in women. The corresponding figures for the United States are 90 per cent and 80 per cent.

Passive or Environmental Smoking

Everybody has had the experience of walking into a smoke-filled room. The coughing and smarting of the eyes that can result is leading many people to ask whether this kind of 'passive' smoking may produce the same sort of serious diseases as those seen in smokers themselves. This possibility has been examined in a number of ways. The most obvious method was to look at the occurrence of smoking-related diseases in the husbands or wives of smokers. Studies of this kind were done in the early 1980s and some involved tens of thousands of people. Epidemiologists used both the case-control and the cohort methods of study that were discussed in Chapter 3. All of these studies were brought together in 1986 by Professor Nicholas Wald and his colleagues in an influential paper published in the *British Medical Journal*. They added together the results of thirteen epidemiological studies and concluded that there was sufficient agreement between them to conclude that there was significant increased risk of lung cancer for someone married to a smoker. The average effect of a married man or woman smoking would be to increase the risk to the non-smoking partner by about 35 per cent. Much controversy remains, because others have suggested that there might have been biases in these studies. It has, for example, been suggested that a non-smoker, when married to a smoker, is more likely to have been given the occasional cigarette during married life and that the explanation of the increased risk might lie in this. This possibility is difficult to reject.

Another approach comes from the laboratory, where work has been done to measure the products of smoking in the urine of non-smokers. These studies show only a few things with any certainty. Products of smoking are to be found in the urine of non-smokers who are married to smokers. Whether there is enough of them to be responsible for an increased risk of lung cancer is not proven.

This controversy is likely to continue and complete resolution is unlikely. We would agree with Sir Richard Doll's view that 'the one conclusion that can be drawn with certainty is that reached by the International Agency for Research on Cancer (in 1986): namely, that the presence of several known laboratory carcinogens in environmental smoke, combined with the knowledge that tobacco actively smoked causes lung cancer in humans, must lead to the presumption that environmental smoke causes some risk of the disease. To this I would add that the risk is unlikely to be greater than that estimated from the epidemiological studies reviewed by Wald' (Doll, 1990).

It is worth setting this risk in perspective. A non-smoking woman has about one chance in 10,000 of getting lung cancer in any year. If she is married to a smoker her chance increases to about one and a half in 10,000 in each year. It might be argued that the consequences for her of her husband's possible lung cancer, which might be as high as 20 in 10,000 in every year, is even worse than the risk to herself. She should try to stop him smoking, but rather more for his sake than for hers.

Risks to *children* in households where parents smoke are real. The Royal College of Physicians in its recent book *Smoking and the Young* reported that children who have smoking parents receive the same amount of nicotine as if they smoked 60–150 cigarettes each year. This is damaging: **the children of parents who smoke are shorter, have twice as much asthma, twice as many chest infections, have more time off school, get more chronic bronchitis and are more likely to die** than the children of non-smokers.

There are many reasons, apart from the cancer risk, for not smoking in the home.

OTHER CAUSES OF LUNG CANCER

Ideas about the cause of lung cancer have been so dominated by recognition of the effect of smoking for the last forty years that it is sometimes easy to forget that there may be other important causal factors and that lung cancer still occurs in non-smokers. The effect of smoking is so strong that it can be quite difficult to unravel other causes, because the presence of a few smokers in any group will so alter the statistics. However, there are undoubtedly other factors at work in the development of lung cancer and many of them can now be judged.

Cooking with a Wok and Rape-seed Oil

Among women who do not smoke lung cancer is commonest in the Chinese. The risk is quite substantial: between two and three times greater than the risk in white women and Japanese women. The effect is observed whether the Chinese live in Shanghai, Hong Kong or Hawaii, and it is limited to women – Chinese non-smoking men have the same chance of lung cancer as a non-smoking white man.

A probable explanation for this observation was unravelled by Gao and colleagues in 1987. It seems that very-high-temperature cooking using some kinds of oil in a wok, and presumably inhaling the burnt chemicals given off, may be a factor in lung cancer. The comparison was made between Chinese women who cooked with rape-seed oil and noted irritation of their eyes when they were cooking and those who never had such irritation and used only soya-bean oil. The difference in lung cancer risk was threefold. Studies in the laboratory show that the fumes from rape-seed oil are more capable of altering DNA (being mutagenic) than are those from soya-bean oil, so the story seems to add up.

This effect is considerably greater than the effect of passive smoking but has not attracted so much attention. Fortunately simple precautions can be taken; improved ventilation in Eastern kitchens might well be achieved without great cost.

Occupation

Once suspicion has been cast on an occupation it is a relatively straightforward, although laborious, task to examine the risk by comparing the incidence of lung cancer in workers in that occupation with that of the general population, and then doing more detailed work to look at the effect of the number of years spent in the occupation or the dose of the suspected agent to which the workers are exposed. Occupational hazard of lung cancer has been shown to be present for workers with asbestos, chrome, hydrocarbon chemicals in the old-style coke and gas industries, some chemicals used in the paint industry and for those who mine uranium (who are probably affected by radon gas from the rocks). New and effective regulations have been brought in to control these industries and the risks have been substantially reduced or eliminated. Careful monitoring remains necessary. Less certain risks have been suggested for workers with cadmium, nickel and vinyl chloride, and some fibres used in the textile industries, and precautions are now taken in industries based on these substances. Butchers appear to have a very small excess of lung cancer over the level which might be predicted. This is entirely unexplained and appears to be independent of smoking habits.

Atmospheric Pollution

Passive smoking and the effects of asbestos and industrial

hazards can act through atmospheric pollution to cause lung cancer. General atmospheric pollution by coal smoke was probably not a very important cause of lung cancer, although it may have contributed to some lung cancers in smokers and is discussed in general together with water pollution later in the book.

Radon gas is radioactive and is present in some rocks. Certain geological conditions allow it to be released from the soil and, in some parts of the world, it appears to accumulate with its radioactive products in houses. In the United Kingdom this is most apparent in Devon and Cornwall and in parts of Derbyshire where the concentration of radon gas in houses may be much higher than in the country in general. However, lung cancer is not especially common in Cornwall and the whole question of a relationship between radon and lung cancer is now the subject of careful examination. Studies from Scandinavia and the United States do suggest that there may be a link between background radon concentrations and lung cancer, and if this is confirmed in Britain, some houses may well need specialized ventilation.

Diet

Questions about diet and cancer are usually posed in relation to breast cancer or bowel cancer, but there is certainly one question mark which remains in relation to lung cancer. In 1975 the Scandinavian worker Bjelke reported that, for any given level of smoking, lung cancer was less frequent in men who took large amounts of vitamin A. This report has been followed up by a number of investigators and it appears that the consumption of vitamin A itself may not be important but that the consumption of beta carotene which can be converted into vitamin A may indeed be of some importance. Blood levels of beta carotene tend to be lower in lung cancer patients. The issue of whether beta carotene is helpful in minimizing the risk of lung cancer is now the subject of a formal-intervention study of the kind discussed in Chapter 3. For this purpose, 23,000 American doctors have agreed to enter an experiment in which only half will take beta carotene. Both groups (those taking it and those not taking it) will be followed up over two or three decades. This study will ultimately give us an answer to what is, at present, simply still a question about a tantalizing possibility.

Genetics

Lung cancer is not inherited in any simple way and, in Scandinavia, studies of identical twins have shown that it is smoking that determines any difference in risk of lung cancer. Identical twins have identical genes and if there were a simple relationship between inherited genes and lung cancer, we would expect the incidence of cancer to be the same in identical twins, regardless of any differences which we might find in the smoking habits of each twin in a pair. This is not the case. If one of a pair of twins smokes, the risk of lung cancer in that twin is greater. While, however, there is no simple link between genetic inheritance and the incidence of lung cancer, the fact remains that some non-smokers get cancer and some smokers do not. This raises the possibility that genetic inheritance may be influential in some subtle way and provide at least part of the explanation for this odd fact. One of the teasing questions which biologists now have to tackle is the part played by innate genetic make-up in protecting some smokers from cancer and disposing some non-smokers to the disease. One suggestion that is being studied is that there may be genetic differences in the way in which the body handles the chemicals produced in cigarettes so as to detoxify them. If research along these, or similar, lines produces answers, we shall be able to identify the patients whose genetic make-up puts them at special risk.

Whatever is discovered, it should not be used as an excuse to ignore the simple advice which now covers this subject – **don't smoke**.

SMOKING AND OTHER KINDS OF CANCER

In any discussion of tobacco smoking and cancer, it is the effects on the lung that dominate both our statistics and our thinking about the cause of cancer, but in fact smoking is also associated with substantial increases in cancer in other organs. Cancers in the mouth, upper airways and upper gullet are found with increased frequency in smokers, presumably because of the direct deposition of tar in these areas. However, epidemiological studies have now shown an increase in cancers of the bladder, pancreas and kidney, which are not places in which tar can accumulate. Even so, the International Agency for Research on Cancer believes this increase to be directly linked to smoking. The report from the United States Surgeon General in 1989 included a calculation of the percentage of deaths from these cancers which can be attributed to cigarettes. The figures are daunting. For men in the United States, the percentage of deaths from lung cancer attributable to smoking is 90 per cent, lip and mouth 92 per cent, gullet 78 per cent, bladder 47 per cent, kidney 48 per cent and larynx 81 per cent. The figures are lower for women, but still sobering and impressive. More recent concern extends to leukaemia, cancer of the neck of the womb and cancer of the stomach.

Our surprise that organs that do not meet smoke directly can be so affected by smoking is readily overcome when it is recognized that many of the chemicals in tobacco smoke dissolve in blood, circulate freely and can be detected in the body. The inhalation of cigarette smoke then simply becomes a way of taking chemicals that cause cancer into all parts of the body.

WHAT IS TO BE DONE?

Our recommendations for avoiding these common cancers are easy and obvious. People should avoid smoking and help others to avoid it too. How can this advice be carried forward? We do not pretend that giving up smoking is an easy matter. One of the authors knows only too well how daunting and frustrating the struggle may be. The smoking of a cigarette delivers nicotine to the central nervous system (the brain and the spinal cord) in less than ten seconds, satisfying the chemical dependence of the addict. Smoking is, however, a complex addiction that extends beyond chemical dependence. The psychological 'rewards' enjoyed by the smoker are many and varied.

Older readers of this book may remember a time when all significant episodes in films were punctuated with a cigarette. For them, the act of smoking may well have become associated with high drama and romance, each early puff providing a passport to the glamorous world of their heroes and heroines. Other smokers will have taken up smoking as an act of youthful defiance, to establish their sociability or mark their passage into adulthood. Such early associations may remain deeply embedded in the image which smokers have of themselves.

Once started, the act of smoking can acquire many psychologically rewarding associations with particular settings or circumstances, which then serve in their turn to trigger the act of smoking. Once it is learned, for example, that smoking a cigarette with a cup of coffee at the end of a good meal is accompanied by feelings of well-being and relaxation, any cup of coffee may become a signal to smoke. Smoking can also become associated with relief from anxiety. A cigarette then becomes a prop in any stressful situation, if only to provide something to do with the hands.

The problem for the smoker who wants to stop for sensible health reasons is that the more distant danger of cancer at a future date seems much less compelling than the immediate pleasures and psychological rewards that he or she gets from today's quota of cigarettes.

Research has shown that public-information programmes on the risks of smoking do not, by themselves, persuade many people to stop smoking. Individuals may either try to avoid the information if they find it threatening or, even if they accept it, fail to accept its relevance to their own circumstances. They will point, for example, to the fact that non-smokers get cancer and that not all smokers succumb to the disease, persuading themselves that they may be in that happy category of people who will escape the risks and be able to puff away into a ripe old age.

In the final analysis, people have to be motivated by an individual need or desire to stop smoking. It has been established that the great majority of those who have given up smoking have done so on their own, without assistance from professionals in the field of health care. Support from family, friends and colleagues, or membership of a support group of other smokers who are trying to give up the habit, will undoubtedly help. Individuals in a support group are understanding of their common problem and can reinforce one another's need and desire to stop smoking.

The recognition that smoking involves an acquired response to particular settings or circumstances can also help those who wish to break the habit. They will realize that, although they may associate cigarettes with pleasant cups of coffee or alcoholic drinks, or with feelings of relief from anxiety in particular settings, they do not, as a rule, even wish to smoke in other situations. They can, for example, survive quite happily without the urge to light up in church or in other settings that have never been associated with smoking. Some people who are trying to give up smoking find it helpful to keep track of the number of cigarettes smoked each day and of their situation and mood at the time each is smoked. In this way, they can build up a picture of the associations which need to be broken. Learned associations can be unlearned, though this may still require a great effort of will.

Nicotine substitutes, such as nicotine chewing-gum or nicotine 'patches' may be helpful to heavy smokers who recognize the risks to their health and wish to stop smoking. Such substitutes work by providing a limited intake of nicotine to minimize withdrawal symptoms while cutting out exposure to the damaging chemicals in smoke.

Those who are near to despair about ever being able to give up smoking should be encouraged by the obvious, but often overlooked, fact that they can get through the night without a cigarette. They should also draw comfort from the knowledge that many people who have failed at the first attempt have ultimately succeeded. People smoke for many different reasons and the strategies which they adopt to stop smoking must take those reasons into account.

If, in the final analysis, people are unable to stop smoking, they should smoke low-tar cigarettes, as the trend towards low tar may already be having a valuable effect in reducing the incidence of lung cancer.

Children and Smoking

Perhaps efforts to prevent smoking should focus even more emphatically on reaching young people before they develop the addiction. Getting the message across to young people will depend on early education and an early focus on 'educating the educators' and support for teachers. Time and money are essential elements in this equation. Many organizations in the United Kingdom and elsewhere in Europe have produced packages for education in schools which have been shown to be effective in increasing knowledge and fostering positive attitudes towards avoiding cancers by avoiding smoking.

Quite a lot is known about children and smoking. Goddard carried out a survey among secondary-school children in 1988 and there has been extensive work by many researchers, notably Dr Ann Charlton for the Cancer Research Campaign. A useful survey is 'Children and Smoking – Your Questions Answered, Cancer Research Campaign 1989'. The first cigarettes are usually taken between the ages of nine and twelve and regular smoking starts as young as eleven in some children. How many regular smokers are there among children? The survey suggests that, among boys, the figures are 2 per cent of twelve-year-olds, 5 per cent of thirteen-year-olds, 8 per cent of fourteen-year-olds and 17 per cent of fifteen-year-olds. The figures are similar in girls but are in fact higher at the age of fourteen, and at fifteen, 22 per cent of girls are regular smokers. During the 1980s there was a small but distinct downward trend in schoolchildren's smoking.

What makes children smoke? Dr Charlton's survey showed that girls are more likely to smoke than boys and that children are more likely to become smokers if one or both parents smoke, if their best friend smokes and if they are unaware of the health risks. Some children still believe that smoking gives people confidence, calms their nerves and controls their weight. Children who smoke are also more likely to drink alcohol, sniff glue, try drugs, go to discos, dislike sports and be low achievers academically and physically.

Education is the answer and can be made more effective by vivid illustrative technology like carbon monoxide monitors. These show clearly that a smoker's exhaled breath contains a lot more carbon monoxide than that of a non-smoker. This gas displaces oxygen from the blood, making it harder for the blood to carry oxygen to muscles and therefore reducing the energy a person has. The monitors can help most impressively to jolt children into an awareness of this risk.

Governments and Economics

What cannot be done by individuals and educators may in some measure be done by governments. We cannot advocate that tobacco should be made illegal. Experience from the prohibition of alcohol in the United States in the 1920s suggests that prohibition of smoking would be costly and futile. Restrictions on advertising and increased taxation to gradually price cigarettes out of the market would be more logical. The trend towards the prohibition of smoking in public vehicles and public buildings should certainly be encouraged. Smokers may grumble as the territory for their habit is reduced and may, perhaps understandably, react in a defiant way if prohibitions are introduced to the accompaniment of hectoring comments on their filthy, dangerous and self-destructive habit, but they usually adapt fairly quickly to the fact that a particular setting can no longer be associated with smoking.

There are many factors which work against the effective reduction in cigarette smoking. A good example of one such factor was given in a study recently published by Dr Warner and colleagues from the United States in the *New England Journal of Medicine*. They analysed 'cigarette advertising and magazine coverage of the hazards of smoking'. They found strong evidence that magazines that carried cigarette advertising tended to have fewer articles on the hazards of smoking. This was particularly true for magazines directed at women. This shows very starkly how uncontrolled cigarette advertising can not only have the direct effect of reducing the likelihood of people stopping smoking but can also indirectly inhibit the spread of knowledge about the hazards of smoking.

Although in northern European countries there is an identified downward trend in smoking, particularly among professionals, this is much less marked in the southern European countries. In 1985, 64 per cent of Spanish physicians smoked and one third of these said they did not consider it of any importance to set a good example to their patients. In the United Kingdom doctors and teachers are not doing badly but nurses have not done well at all and were in fact increasing their rate of smoking until very recently.

In 1992, the Department of Health in the United Kingdom produced a document called 'The Health of the Nation'. It included as an objective the reduction of death and ill health from cancers and acknowledged that tobacco use accounted for around 30 per cent of all cancer deaths. Those who produced this policy on health acknowledged that a reduction in smoking would depend on a number of measures, including health education, health promotion, new policies in the workplace and controls on advertising.

Currently, some 33 per cent of men and 30 per cent of women in the United Kingdom smoke cigarettes. The number is falling and is predicted to be of the order of 25 per cent by the year 2000. The new health policies include a commitment to try to reduce the proportion of people who smoke cigarettes to 22 per cent of men and 21 per cent of women by the year 2000. If even this modest goal can be achieved there should be a major impact on lung cancer deaths and the many other tobacco-related cancers.

More powerful and pervasive economic forces are also at work. The case against smoking is overwhelmingly strong and a large reduction in mortality from many important cancers would be brought about if we could eradicate the habit of smoking within the European Community. The health departments of the member countries are active on the anti-smoking front and the Europe against Cancer campaign has been particularly energetic in organizing campaigns against smoking. There are many reasons why such campaigns are not having a dramatic impact, and we have already touched on some of these.

However, few people are aware that the European Community actually subsidizes the growing of tobacco. When the subsidy was introduced, tobacco growing was confined to parts of Italy and small areas of France and Germany, and the amounts of subsidy were relatively small. The effects of the subsidy were to stimulate a massive increase in tobacco growing in those countries and to encourage a shift towards tobacco production in Spain and Greece as they prepared to join the Community. A recent editorial article in the *European Journal of Cancer Prevention* points out that tobacco takes 3.75 per cent of the EC agricultural subsidies, making tobacco the single most subsidized product. It is ironic to say the least that the subsidy for tobacco production is two or three times the budget for the Europe against Cancer campaign. Those concerned with devising European agricultural policy have an understandable interest in the economic welfare of European farmers. We doubt, however, whether tobacco production is essential for Europe when tobacco is killing so many Europeans.

We must acknowledge that some poorer countries in the less developed parts of the world are highly dependent on tobacco production to boost their export earnings and that there is no doubt that a worldwide decline in demand for tobacco would have a serious effect on their economies unless they were able to switch to other highly saleable crops. This is not the case for Europe, however. The editors of the *European Journal of Cancer Prevention* have suggested that those responsible for EC agricultural policy would do better to switch their subsidies away from tobacco production into efforts to promote the production and consumption of fresh fruit and vegetables.

The picture is equally depressing if we consider the policies of the governments of some member states in the European Community. In Italy, the government has a monopoly on the purchase of locally grown tobacco and on the production of cigarettes from that tobacco. The governments of Spain and Greece have similar financial interests in locally grown tobacco. As the *European Journal of Cancer Prevention* points out, 'These governments therefore have a financial interest in their nationals *not* giving up smoking.'

The Association of European Cancer Leagues published in 1992 a document called *Europe's Public Health Scandal: A Critique of European Community Tobacco Subsidies*. We quote here the conclusion to their report:

> Most tobacco production in the European Community would be untenable without artificial prices being guaranteed to producers and growers and financed by revenue from largely unwitting taxpayers. The subsidy regime has developed into a panacea for disadvantaged remote rural areas rather than a rational commodity support. It is based on an unessential, non-food crop which, where it can be marketed to European palates at EC prices, erodes the health of the Community, and where it cannot, requires gigantic export subsidies to reach poor developing countries who can ill afford additional bought-in mortality. Tobacco subsidies help to damage the lives of consumers across the world, their families, and the economy of their own countries. By dispassionate standards, this cannot be rated as a very intelligent deployment of resources, or a solution to the long-term problems of rural disadvantage. By compassionate standards, it can only be judged a policy disaster of tragic proportions.

On 15 May 1992 European Community health ministers met to discuss a ban on the advertising of tobacco. They postponed a decision! The next week saw publication of the report by a World Health Organization consultative group on statistical aspects of smoking-related mortality from Richard Peto and colleagues in the *Lancet* on 23 May 1992; the report concluded that

About one fifth of the people now living in developed countries (i.e. about one quarter of one billion out of one and a quarter billion) will, on current smoking patterns, eventually be killed by tobacco, losing an average of about fifteen years of life expectancy per death.

Elsewhere the epidemic is generally at an earlier stage but recent large increases in cigarette use in countries such as China means that tobacco will, in a few decades, also become one of the most important causes of premature death in less developed countries.

5
Diet and Cancer

There are many facets to the relationship between diet and cancer. We have to consider whether people's food intake is an important factor in determining their risk of getting cancer of any kind. This is perhaps the primary question and it is the one upon which we will concentrate in this book. There are, however, other questions, and the second is whether altering the diet once a patient is diagnosed as having cancer will affect the outcome. The third question is whether altering diet during the period of treatment of cancer can improve a patient's well-being and quality of life. The three questions have to be tackled separately. Factors influencing cancer causation are unlikely to be the same as those that influence either the progression of the disease once it is established or the patient's well-being during treatment. The biology of cancer is one of steady and progressive change, as discussed in Chapter 2, and the things which influence cancer very early in its course are likely to be different from the things that influence it at a later stage.

Although we shall concentrate on diet as a possible cause of cancer, it is worth making a few comments on the relationship between diet on the one hand and the progress of an established cancer and the patient's well-being during treatment for that cancer on the other hand. It is clear from a wealth of clinical experience that patients who pay careful attention to their diet feel better during treatment for their cancer and that they gain a great deal of satisfaction from the control that this gives them over at least one very important aspect of their lives. The quality of their lives is better when they ensure a balanced intake of protein and calories (often with vitamin supplements) once cancer is established and once they are undergoing treatments. To this extent, diet is an important element in the management of the illness. However, although quite a lot of research work has been done on this topic and very many claims have been made, there is no good evidence that major modifications of diet will lead to people living longer. This is a controversial subject because of its implications for practitioners of 'alternative medicine', who sometimes advocate relatively extreme diets. It is not the purpose of this chapter to enter that controversy – our focus is on prevention.

The relationship between cancer cause, cancer prevention and diet is in itself pretty controversial. Great excitement has been generated by a number of experimental observations, and many people hold strong views on this topic. It seems very reasonable to speculate that diet will be an important determinant of cancer because it is such a large part of our environment. Through our diet we take in complex mixtures, and consume literally thousands of chemicals every day. Some of these are well known and well characterized scientifically and others are not so fully understood. Many of the important cancers occur in the gastro-intestinal tract which involves tissues extending from the mouth through the gullet (oesophagus), stomach, small intestine and large intestine to the rectum. These tissues, with the exception of the small intestine, are prone to cancers and it does seem likely that the food with which they have continuous contact is likely to be an element in causing these cancers.

It is a great leap from this theory to any precise idea of how far and in what ways it may be true. What particular elements in food are important and, perhaps more importantly, what conscious changes in diet might be acceptable and beneficial in actually reducing the incidence of cancer? Scientists, in association with government agencies, the food industry and a number of pressure groups, have been working on this problem for decades. It is one of the most difficult areas within which to unravel fact from speculation and it is beset by great difficulty in performing the necessary studies. Suspecting that food can be an important element in cancer cause is one thing; proving it is another; pinpointing elements in the diet that are guilty and can be eliminated from it by realistic and acceptable measures is yet another.

There is one question which it is important to touch on before we go on to discuss what is known and what is speculative. This has to do with the practicalities of suggesting dietary changes that will affect a large proportion of the population when, in fact, only a minority of the population will get a particular cancer. At present it is very difficult to predict who that minority will be. If therefore one suggests sweeping dietary changes, the majority may make such changes and gain nothing by them. For this reason, enthusiasts must be very cautious before suggesting extreme changes in diet for everyone. The argument was put very well by Dr Michael Hill in 1985 at a European conference on diet and cancer.

> Cancer of the large bowel [large intestine] is one of the most common cancers in the Western world. About 5 per cent of us will get it. Consequently 95 per cent of us will not. We do not know in advance who is who. Giving advice therefore implies giving advice to the whole population. We know of a fairly large number of risk factors for colon cancer and fairly profound changes in the diet should be recommended. Apart from the effect on the society and the production of foodstuff, this also has the drawback that 95 per cent of the population make these changes completely in vain, since they are not going to get colon cancer anyhow.

> We should therefore be able to tell them with great confidence that this change in diet does in no way imply an increased risk of acquiring other ailments or perhaps other cancers. Since this is definitely true and obvious for colon cancer, which is a common cancer, it is of course even more so for all other cancers.

While, however, we should heed this sensible note of caution, we must also recognize that the overall impact of dietary change on the cancer problem in total could be very substantial. Sir Richard Doll, in an influential article written in 1981, attempted to estimate the proportion of cancer that might be due to factors, single or multiple, in the diet. This was an elaborate epidemiological exercise which, as he would be the first to admit, required many assumptions. The estimates were very difficult to make and had to be judged on the basis of variations in cancer incidence between different populations with different diets which might or might not be finally proven to be important causes of cancer. Making allowances for the guesswork involved, Doll estimated that the proportion of cancers which are due to diet lie somewhere between 10 and 70 per cent. Two things about this estimate are daunting. First, the magnitude of the problem is brought home. Second, the difficulty of the estimation is very clear. Since that paper was written we have learned a great deal more about the causes of cancer and the relationship to diet, and we are more certain of a few things.

At the end of this chapter we shall make some recommendations and allow ourselves some speculation. We will concentrate now on a critical look at how the information on diet and cancer is gained, and just how convincing it is.

What Do We Eat?

That diets vary between countries is obvious. The main source of carbohydrate may be rice or potatoes and some populations may be vegetarian while others may live largely on meat or fish. Within a country, there may be smaller but equally important variations. It is therefore difficult to talk about the average diet. The average Western woman was said in one American study in the mid-1980s to consume about 1,600

Calories of energy per day with 70 g of protein, 70 g of fat, 170 g of carbohydrate and 3–4 g of crude fibre. Within the vitamin intake, the daily average for vitamin C was 107 mg and the average for vitamin A about 5,000 international units. The problem for researchers lies not only in estimating what an individual takes in but in getting some idea of how much variation there is. For the main constituents of the diet, the proteins, fats and carbohydrates, most people will fall within 20 per cent of the average for the population. For the parts of the diet that are small in quantity but are of vital importance the variation may be greater. A good example is vitamin A, where the scatter is very wide, and this variation is not only between people but between one day and another for the same person. One statistic might serve to illustrate this point. Someone studying dietary vitamin A might expect with reasonable confidence to be able to gain information on the vitamin A intake of an individual by studying that person's diet. However, the variation from day to day means that one single day's observation might not be very close to that person's average. How many days of observation are necessary to get close to that average? Willett, an eminent American working in this field, has calculated the number of days of observation which are necessary to achieve a confident estimation of vitamin A intake. If you want to be confident that you have an estimate that is within 10 per cent of the average for that person you need to continue assessing vitamin A intake for 424 days! If you want to be confident that you are within 40 per cent of the person's average you need twenty-six days. Not a terribly precise business. Fortunately, for other elements in diet, like dietary fat, the variation is a lot less and fourteen days of checks will get you to within 20 per cent of the average. Estimating fibre content is notoriously difficult and there is still argument about what is meant by 'fibre'.

In addition to the main features of a diet (the fat, the

carbohydrate and the protein) and to the minerals and vitamins that we also take in, there are many other substances which go to make up the total content of a diet. *Additives* are added to food for preservation or colouring or flavouring. They are a small element of the food but have attracted a great deal of concern. They are in fact the best scientifically understood and regulated of the minor constituents of our food. *Agricultural additives* include pesticides, fungicides, herbicides and hormones for plants and animals, and again they are a small part of our diet but are quite properly a source of great concern. *Microbe contaminants* arise from all sorts of things which can grow on food, perhaps particularly in the form of moulds, and we do know that at least one mould product, a substance called aflatoxin, may be a factor in some human cancers in developing countries. There is not, however, much evidence for the direct relationship between this mould and cancer in the developed world. *Chemicals formed in cooking* are many and varied, particularly when cooking involves high temperatures, as in the example of wok cookery mentioned in Chapter 4. Studies in the laboratory show that even the act of heating meat without necessarily burning it can generate lots of chemicals which, when tested in the laboratory, are capable of causing mutagens (altering the DNA). Whether these have anything to do with human cancer is unclear. Finally, any diet will contain many *other natural substances* which are made by the plants and animals that we consume. All plants and animal cells have constituents which are crucial for their own survival and which are consumed when they are eaten. Plants may, for example, contain chemically complicated toxins (poisons) which serve to protect them against insects.

As we have said, the main constituents of diet in terms of quantity are fat, protein and carbohydrate. These are often referred to in discussions about diet and deemed to be either 'good' or 'bad'. In fact, they are all essential parts of what we eat and the real question focuses on how much of each is best.

Carbohydrate

Carbohydrate is mainly an energy source. It is moderately rich in energy and we get about 4 Calories out of every gram of carbohydrate. The big contributors of carbohydrate in Western diets are bread and potatoes, although carbohydrates are part of every living cell and there will be some present in almost everything that we eat. If we eat too much carbohydrate, it can be converted and stored as fat and can therefore be one of the factors that causes obesity. The form in which we take our carbohydrate may influence its value. If, for example, carbohydrates are taken in combination with fibre in the form of bran then they may be important to our health. In the process of digestion, carbohydrates are broken down into smaller elements (sugar molecules) which can be more easily absorbed. There is a wide range of different sugars and the value of each is still the subject of some debate.

Protein

Proteins are the building bricks of living organisms and they are many and varied. Different protein structures are largely responsible for the shape, structure and function of the biological systems which make up living things. Proteins form the structures which make up the internal frame within which the contents of the cells are found. They are responsible for the movement in muscle cells which create our power; and the very many complicated chemical processes that occur within cells are all controlled by proteins called enzymes. Each different protein has an individual structure and is made up of a long string of smaller molecules called amino acids. The sequence of the amino acids is determined by the genetic code discussed in Chapter 2. Once the sequence is in place the protein will take up a particular shape and be folded in various ways to allow it to carry out its role. In general, when we eat proteins we break them down in the process of digestion in the gut into amino acids and we need to take in large quantities of amino acid for our own rebuilding processes in the cells and tissues of our bodies. If we have surplus amino acids we can use them as energy and they are a rich source of energy, about as rich as carbohydrate.

Fat

Fats have had something of a bad press. The association between fat intake and obesity is a pretty obvious one and is real because fats are a very high energy source. There is more than twice as much energy in a gram of fat as there is in a gram of carbohydrate or protein. We use fats for storing energy and hence lay them down in our bodies in places which are sometimes all too obvious. We also use particular fats for particular purposes like building the membranes that make up the outer coats of cells. In particular, some vitamins, including vitamins A, D, E and K, are soluble in fats and not in water, so we get most of them by taking in fatty foods. Fats may be saturated (this term referring to the relationship of the carbon and the hydrogen in their structure) and such fats tend to be found in animal sources, or they may be unsaturated, in which case they will tend to be found in vegetable sources. A great deal of attention has been paid to the fat content of diet as a possible causative factor in cancer.

Why is it so Difficult to Study Diet and Cancer?

Every attempt to unravel the relationship between diet and cancer runs up against a whole series of difficulties.

- *Diet is very complex*. We have already made it clear how

many different factors there are in the average diet. Not only is it always going to be difficult to work out which factors are important but we must recognize that they are not likely to act independently. A diet that is rich in something that causes cancer might not seem too bad if it is also rich in something which gives protection against cancer. Unravelling the interactions between these factors presents real problems.

- *It is difficult to measure diet accurately*. Not only is there great variation in diet but people make a lot of mistakes in recalling their food intake over the previous days. In some studies as many as 50 per cent of people will be found to have made a mistake about important dietary elements when these are cross-checked against independent observations of what they have actually eaten. For some reason, fruit and vegetable content seems to be particularly vulnerable to errors of recall.

- *It is difficult to know the amount of a nutrient in any item eaten*. For instance, if you have a steak, how much fat is there likely to be in it? This will vary from animal to animal and depends on the preparation and method by which it is cooked. Some of these variations are moderate for the minor constituents of diet. For instance, the variation in carotene, an important constituent of many vegetables, can be two- or threefold between different vegetables. Essentially the more orange a carrot is, the more carotene it contains. Two- or threefold variations may not be crucial in working out the quantities of a substance in someone's diet but other factors in the diet may vary several hundredfold. Selenium is an element which has been associated with a protective effect against cancers in some studies. The selenium content of a food will depend upon the selenium content of the soil upon which the vegetables were grown or the animals grazed.

Selenium can vary between such low levels that animals are at risk of selenium deficiency through to such high levels that animals are at risk of selenium poisoning. The selenium content of meat may vary two hundredfold and, for most dietary histories, the source of a particular food may not be known. It can be seen that dietary histories that are taken in an attempt to estimate selenium intake are not likely to be worthwhile, and other approaches to this topic have had to be found.

- *Laboratory experiments are difficult to interpret*. The impact of diet on cells grown in laboratory dishes is not easy to work out and if we observe the impact of changing the nutrient fluid in which the cells are suspended such observations will only give us weak clues as to what we might expect from any changes in exposure for these kinds of cells in a person. Observations on rats and mice which are fed on diets with differing contents of, for instance, fat or vitamins have given us some clues. However, the diets of small animals cannot accurately reflect what happens in people. Information from experiments may contribute a little piece to the jigsaw as we try to build the truth about the relationship between diet and cancer but they will never be capable of giving us clear answers.

- *Epidemiological studies are hard to perform on diet*. Case control and cohort studies of the kind which we discussed earlier are difficult because it is hard to estimate exactly people's exposure to different risks in the diet. Nevertheless, they can be done and they have been undertaken for many important dietary factors. The greatest difficulty for the epidemiologist is that he or she cannot easily do the intervention studies that may be most informative. Any intervention study can only be conducted with the consent of a very large number of people and those people then need to stick quite well to the rules within the study. Major change in diet is hard enough to achieve even for a compelling personal reason like obesity. It is that much more difficult for the sake of a scientific study. The individual people involved cannot be absolutely certain that the changes in the diet are going to benefit them. Smaller dietary changes like adding supplements in the form of capsules or tablets may be possible and it is in this area that most progress has been made.

SPECIFIC ASPECTS OF DIET

No blanket statement about any connection between diet and cancer is possible. The topic has to be broken up into a number of areas. It would be unwise to attempt to be comprehensive or to include any analysis of claims for particular narrowly focused diets. Diets which consist exclusively of grapes or carrots or lean red meat may have their advocates but they are never going to be to the taste of a large proportion of the population and may carry their own risks. We believe that the examination of our knowledge about diet has to focus on things which are achievable and reasonable, bearing in mind that a big change in diet for the whole population will only benefit those members of that population who were ultimately destined to get a cancer. We also have to concentrate on those areas where there is much useful knowledge. For many of the more extreme diets that have been advocated so little real knowledge exists and the suggestions are so speculative that we cannot concentrate on them in a book which is intended to bring scientific knowledge into focus for the interested layman.

We have chosen to concentrate on the following:

1. *Dietary fat*. This is a particularly important consideration in relation to breast cancer and gastro-intestinal cancers.

2. *Dietary fibre and starch*. This is particularly crucial in any

discussion of the cause of cancer of the lower intestine or bowel.

3. *Dietary vitamins and minerals, in particular vitamins A and E and selenium*. There has been a wealth of studies of these and some speculative conclusions are possible since a great number of the studies have been sufficiently encouraging to prompt further scientific work that is being conducted all over the world at the moment.

4. *Chemical additives and cooking*. Materials produced by cooking and additives have to be considered, although any very general statement is difficult to make because of the huge number of chemicals to consider.

5. *Obesity*.

6. *Alcohol*.

1. Fat

The intake of fat (and particularly animal fats) has been put forward as an important causative factor in breast cancer. The story starts with comparisons made between the fat intake of individuals in particular countries and deaths from breast cancer in those countries. We have tried to show the results of these observations in Figure 12, plotting the countries of the world by the fat content in their diet and against the incidence of breast cancer. Detailed statistics are not necessary to demonstrate that countries with a high fat intake in the diet are also those where breast cancer is common. Other studies show that the association is mainly with saturated animal fat in the diet. At first glance, this is strong evidence, and indeed it is important and cannot be ignored but it does not prove that there is a link between dietary fat and breast cancer.

The information on fat consumption in these countries is

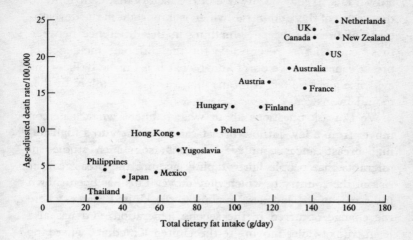

Figure 12 Dietary fat and breast cancer.

(Prepared from data provided by the Cancer Research Campaign.)

not very precise. It tends to be what is known as 'disappearance data'. The fats enter the food distribution system and disappear from it. That means a lot of them will have been eaten but that some will have been cut off and thrown away. More importantly, this link is an *association* and not necessarily a *causation*. Going back to the argument that we considered when we talked about the work of epidemiologists, it will be recognized that this distinction is a very important one indeed. There are many differences between the countries on that list. In general, the rich countries have a high fat intake with lots of meat and the poor countries have a lower fat intake because their diet is generally less rich. In fact the link between gross national product and breast cancer is almost as strong as the link to animal fats. It may be any one of the factors that contribute to the wealth of these countries which is important in the development of breast cancer. Something in the difference between these countries is responsible for the different incidence of breast cancer but we don't know what it is on the basis of the evidence given so far. It means that we have to explore further to find an answer.

We can ask questions about what happens when a person moves from a low-fat/low-breast-cancer country to a high-fat/high-breast-cancer country. It seems from such studies of migrants that people fairly rapidly acquire the breast cancer risk of the country to which they move. This has been shown to be true of the Japanese moving to the United States, where the change occurred in the second generation, and has also been true of Poles moving to the United Kingdom, where the change appeared in the first generation. Again, this suggests that something is happening in those high-fat/high-breast-cancer countries, but it doesn't mean that the important factor will be the fat in the diet. It could be any one of the many other differences between those countries. If we look at special populations who have a low risk of breast cancer, like the Seventh Day Adventists religious group in the high-risk United States, we find that they have a low fat and low meat intake but that there are many other socio-economic differences between that group and other people in the States.

Where else can we look for clues? We can look at changes over time in different countries. Japan gives us an opportunity here because there has been a dramatic increase in the fat content of the Japanese diet in the last three decades. It may not be that hamburgers and chips have completely displaced the traditional diet of rice and fish, but there has been something of a move in that direction. The increase in breast cancer in Japan remains quite small so far, which perhaps argues against dietary fat as a causative factor. We must, however, remember that the relationship in time of changing fat intake to change in breast cancer incidence is unknown, and we have already mentioned that when people move to countries of known high risk it may take one or even two generations before the change is seen.

We find that studying the patterns of breast cancer in different countries and trying to link them to the patterns of fat consumption has given some pointers for further research but has not produced conclusive results. Articles are still written which point to the associations which have been found and which, quite unjustifiably, proceed to make the assumption that we should all eat less fat. There may be good reasons for advocating less fat in our diets but the evidence based on the differences between countries for breast cancer risk is not conclusive.

At this point we have to move on to the second stage of the epidemiological research process which we described in Chapter 3. This is the stage of *analytical epidemiology*. Here we are talking about the case-control, cohort and intervention studies and a large number of these have been performed. In case-control studies patients with breast cancer are asked about their dietary fat and a group of control subjects who do not have breast cancer but who are matched in other ways to the patients are asked the same questions. The two are then compared. Such studies have been undertaken carefully in Canada, the United States and Australia. Argument rages around them but it has to be said that the findings were essentially negative. That is to say, no consistent difference was found between the fat intake of breast cancer patients and the fat intake of other people in the population in these studies.

What about the cohort studies? The reader will recall that in this approach groups of people are identified and the dietary fat history is taken. They are then followed over a long period of time to see who gets breast cancer and to find out if there is any connection with their dietary fat intake as measured at the beginning of the study. Three large studies of this kind have been published during the 1980s. In the United States, the Seventh Day Adventists were followed for twenty-one years. Again in the United States, 89,538 nurses aged between thirty-four and fifty-nine were followed up after giving a dietary history. In a smaller US study over five thousand women were followed up. These were immensely difficult studies to perform and required a big logistic effort. Again it has to be said that the results were essentially negative. No link was found between dietary fat and breast cancer in the cohort studies.

Ideally, the whole question could be resolved by an intervention study in which some women would agree to reduce their dietary fat substantially while others would not, and we could then see if there was a reduction in the breast cancer incidence in those who had reduced their fat. It has been argued that this should be done, but no such study has been undertaken. Preliminary work has suggested that it might be possible but that it would be a hugely expensive and very time-consuming effort, with large numbers of people having to make substantial changes in their diet. Until the kind of information that we would get from an intervention study is available we will not have a certain answer, but, in our opinion, the balance of the evidence at present is rather against a strong link between dietary fat and breast cancer.

The studies of differences between countries in fat intake and incidence of breast cancer seem to point in one direction, although not conclusively. The case-control studies and cohort studies seem to point in the opposite direction. How can we explain this?

One response to this is to say that the situation is not really confused. A perfectly consistent explanation for all the observations would be that there is no causative link between dietary fat and breast cancer. The case-control studies and the cohort studies by the analytical epidemiologists are negative and this is in keeping with this view. The comparisons between countries do not prove a causative link, they just show that there is an association and there may be another explanation that we have not yet uncovered.

It is, however, probably premature to conclude that there is no causative link at all between fat intake and breast cancer, and there are a number of reasons for remaining cautious and open minded. The first relates to the range of dietary variation. The analytical epidemiology has been carried out in Western countries and, in general, in such countries, the range of fat intake (expressed as the percentage of total calories taken as fat) is from about 30 to 43 per cent. This is a narrow range. Between different countries of the world, where variations in wealth and dietary traditions are much greater, the range is between 10 and 45 per cent, a much wider spread. This may matter in assessing the results of studies, because when the range of variation is narrow, it is possible for the analytical epidemiologist to miss important links. Just how important this could be has been illustrated by looking at the link between cigarette smoking and lung cancer. Cigarette smoking causes lung cancer. Of that there is no doubt. The full range of cigarette smoking is from no cigarettes at all to a large number of cigarettes each day and if we look over this whole range the evidence for the link between smoking and lung cancer is overwhelmingly strong. People who do not smoke are very much less likely to get lung cancer than those who smoke thirty or more cigarettes a day, and this is perfectly obvious from the statistics. In the jargon of medical researchers, the difference is 'statistically significant'. If, however, we look at differences in incidence of lung cancer between those who smoke fifteen cigarettes a day and those who smoke thirty or more (a much narrower range), the differences are much less striking. In other words, we cannot demonstrate statistically that your prospects are better if you smoke fifteen cigarettes a day than if you smoke thirty or more. This is the effect of having only a narrow range to look at, and it may well be that the range of dietary fat which is typical of Western countries is also too narrow to give us strong statistical evidence that fat intake is associated with the development of breast cancer. We cannot say for certain that this is the reason why epidemiologists have failed to show links to dietary fat in their recent studies, but the possibility has to be borne in mind.

Finally, some experimental studies have been undertaken in the laboratory to see if the diet of mice and rats has led to breast tumours or not. The experiments have been reported to support the fat/breast cancer link but, in fact, they have mostly been studies of the total calorie intake of the animals. Vets have undertaken case-control studies in which dogs who have been found to have breast tumours have been compared for their dietary intake to other dogs who do not have breast tumours. Even these studies have failed to confirm any link between fat and breast cancer.

Fat intake is also discussed in relation to bowel cancer. Like breast cancer, bowel cancer is commoner in wealthy countries and fat intake is high in those countries. So there is an *association* between fat intake and bowel cancer. Is fat a cause? It is not clear. Studies have been undertaken to look at possible links between both fat and meat intake and bowel cancer. The evidence is mixed: for *fat* nine studies claimed to find a link, sixteen said that fat had no effect and two suggested that fat actually protected against bowel cancer. For *meat*, nine studies said meat intake was linked to bowel cancer, twelve said meat had no effect. All pretty uncertain, although the link to cooked-meat intake may be more convincing.

Where does the practical person go from here, in the absence of certainty? We think it is reasonable to look carefully at the fat content of diet and to try to reduce it somewhat, so that of the total amount of calories taken in perhaps only about 30 per cent is taken as fat. We suggest this not only because we are not absolutely sure that there is no link to breast cancer, although that is part of the argument. The better arguments are that fat is a powerful source of obesity because of its high energy content and that fat is implicated in cardiovascular (heart) disease. Modest, acceptable reductions in total fat intake make sense and there are ways of achieving these without making a diet miserable or unpalatable. Smaller quantities of butter, cheese and red meat are at the heart of diets with lower fat intake, and more fruit and vegetables will contribute to a healthier diet. Chicken and fish are low in fat.

2. Fibre and Starch

The relationship between the amount of fibre in the diet and the development of cancers of the large bowel has been much investigated and is probably real. Food fibres are made up of a large group of plant materials with very varying chemical make-up. We often eat the whole plant and this will consist of many components besides fibres. Most fibres remain intact in the bowel and therefore make up the bulk of the stool or faeces. How do fibres work to reduce the risk of cancer? It may just be that a large volume dilutes any other elements in the diet that might place people at risk of cancer or it may be that they have a more subtle effect, through alteration of the acidity of the stool, which, in turn, may alter the activity of chemicals that are placing people at risk of cancer. Starch content in diet has been explored more recently since it was realized that some starch is not digested and reaches the bowel.

How good is the evidence? In the early 1970s the British surgeon Denis Burkitt proposed that dietary fibre might reduce the risk of large bowel cancer, and there have been more than

forty studies designed to assess this proposition epidemiologic-
ally and in the laboratory in the last two decades. In a recent
review of the state of the evidence, it was found that thirty-two
of the forty studies supported the association between a high
fibre intake and a low incidence of cancer in the large bowel.
There is a consistency here that is much clearer than that seen
in the studies relating fat to breast cancer or bowel cancer.
Comparisons between countries show a close association between fibre content in the diet and colon cancer incidence or
mortality. Special populations with a high intake of fibre-rich
food, like Mormons and Seventh Day Adventists in the United
States and Scandinavians in country areas, have a low incidence
of large bowel cancer. Subsequent analytic epidemiology studies and case-control studies have, in general, been positive and
have confirmed an association between dietary fibre and the
risk of large bowel cancer. A few studies have been negative
but the consensus is clear. Animal diets have also been the
subject of investigation and the evidence from these broadly
supports the importance of fibre.

The Scandinavian studies are perhaps particularly important. In Finland the total dietary fat intake, particularly of
saturated fat in dairy products, is similar to that in the United
States, the United Kingdom and several other Western European countries. However, individuals in rural Finland traditionally have a high intake of bran cereal fibre which results in a
considerable stool bulk and more frequent stools. They also
have a low death rate from large bowel cancer, less than half of
that in England and Wales, the United States, Germany and
France, and only a third of that of Denmark.

However, it has been difficult to work out which types of
fibre are the most important. Cereal fibre, such as that found
in wheat bran, seems to be most effective in reducing the risk
of large bowel cancers.

How much fibre should we eat? The average Western man

Table 1
Fibre in Your Diet

Very high fibre (more than 8 g/helping)	Wholemeal bread Beans in tomato sauce Frozen peas Large helping of breakfast bran
High fibre (6–8 g/helping)	Muesli Spinach Raspberries
Moderate fibre (4–6 g/helping)	Granary bread Bran flakes Bananas Wholemeal pasta
Some fibre (less than 2 g/helping)	White bread Porridge Breakfast cereal Carrots Apples and pears Potatoes Brown rice

takes in between 10 and 15 g of fibre per day and a desirable intake if we take the Finns as our model is probably in the order of 20–30 g per day. Such an intake can be achieved fairly readily by a diet that contains a modest increase in fruit and vegetables and perhaps some bran supplements. A number of bran-rich breakfast cereals are now manufactured and a 40–50 g serving for breakfast will contain some 10–15 g of fibre. It would seem wise to consider bran at breakfast time, particularly if it is taken instead of bacon and eggs on occasion. The morale-boosting effect of a bacon and egg breakfast before a busy day should not be underestimated, but it should perhaps become a rare treat.

The starch connection will be harder to work out because much starch is digested in the upper parts of the stomach and only recently has it become clear that some gets through to the bowel. High starch diets are found in countries with low bowel cancer rates and the link is at least as strong as that to fibre. It is too soon to make firm recommendations about the best diet policy – common cereal starches are digested and do not affect the bowel. Banana starches are not digested well and may therefore be a good source of protection. More research is needed on starch and bowel cancer.

3. Vitamins and Minerals

Vitamins are substances which occur naturally within the diet, usually in small quantities. They are essential for normal life and health, and when people are deficient in vitamins specific illnesses result. For instance, vitamin A is necessary for normal function of the eyes and skin; the absence of vitamin C results in scurvy; the numerous B vitamins prevent a range of illnesses from anaemia to skin rashes; and vitamin D is essential for normal calcium levels in the blood and for normal bones. It is also true that, under some circumstances, excessive doses of vitamins can be dangerous. For instance, vitamin D can cause an excess of calcium in the blood which can be damaging in many ways. Too much vitamin A causes liver damage and too much vitamin C can result in kidney stones. Vitamins are therefore necessary for our survival, as well as being potentially damaging when given in excessive doses.

Large doses of vitamins have been used to treat established cancer and are very popular with practitioners of alternative medicine. In general, this is a harmless practice which gives a sense of activity and control to many cancer patients and is therefore beneficial to their quality of life. However, as a small number of carefully performed studies have shown, there is no evidence that treating established cancers with vitamins prolongs people's lives. All that we can say is that a healthy diet with plenty of vitamins is a good idea for all patients with cancer.

Greater interest now centres on whether vitamins can be used in doses above those normally present in the diet to reduce the risk of getting cancer. This subject is highly controversial and has led to some red herrings being pursued in earlier research. However, some sufficiently exciting clues are beginning to emerge for us to take seriously the idea that vitamins may have a role in preventing cancer. The evidence for routine supplementation of the diet with vitamins as a preventative for cancer is not yet sufficiently strong to allow us to make a firm recommendation about vitamin supplements, but we may not be too far from that point. The results of several current studies which should report in a few years' time are likely to be very helpful and probably conclusive.

Vitamin A, Retinoids and Carotene

Most of the research on vitamins in relation to cancer cause has focused on the retinoids. This group of chemicals includes vitamin A (also called retinol), a closely chemically related substance called retinoic acid and some chemically modified versions of this molecule. Carotene is a close relative of vitamin A which is present in carrots and other vegetables, and some of it is converted into vitamin A in the body. Carotene is different from vitamin A not only in the sources from which it can be obtained but also in its handling by the body. Concentrations of vitamin A are carefully controlled in the body whereas concentrations of beta carotene are less precisely controlled.

Vitamin A is an important element in the normal growth, development and function of the cells covering surfaces of the body. These include the skin as the external surface and the lining of the intestine and other internal organs. Vitamin A deficiency in man is not known to be associated with cancer but vitamin A deficiency in animals can be associated with an increase in certain types of cancer and with certain changes in some of the lining tissues which then look as if they might become cancerous.

In laboratory experiments in which cells are kept alive in cultures, vitamin A will alter the appearance and behaviour of cells, shifting them from the behaviour of cancer cells towards the behaviour of normal cells. This observation is not made in all experiments but a substantial number of culture systems have now been studied and the effect is moderately consistent.

Recently, a number of substances closely related to vitamin A have been produced chemically. These are very strong and include so-called cis-retinoic acid, which is capable of causing the regression of cancers in some experiments.

The effects of beta carotene may work in part through its being converted into retinol, but carotene itself is known to be capable of inactivating chemically reactive substances (known as free radicals) within cells and this 'free radical scavenging' might be important in preventing damage to DNA. Overall, the experimental evidence linking vitamin A and its relatives to the development of cancer is sufficient to justify careful examination of the evidence from epidemiology.

In 1975 a Norwegian epidemiologist called Bjelke undertook a postal survey of 8,278 Norwegian men and collected information on their cigarette smoking and their dietary habits. Their vitamin A intake was calculated from answers which they gave to the questionnaire, using tables of the content of typical Norwegian food. Records were kept for five years to see what happened to these men and, in particular, the incidence of lung cancer was studied. In this group of people, those with a higher index of vitamin A intake had a lower incidence of lung cancer and this was true at all levels of cigarette smoking. At least two other groups of people have been used in such studies including those followed up in a large study in America

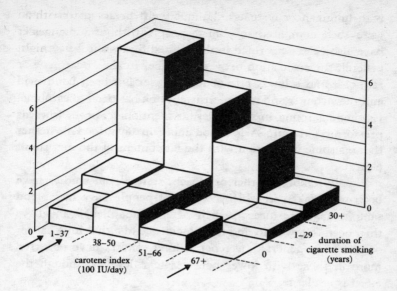

Figure 13 Link between carotene intake, cigarette smoking and lung cancer.

Examine the people who have a high carotene index (67 +, single arrow). Even those who smoke heavily have only a low cancer incidence. Those who have a low carotene index (1–37, double arrows) have a low incidence of lung cancer if they do not smoke. However, if they are heavy smokers the figure is very high – demonstrated by the tall 'skyscrapers' at the back of the diagram.
(From data from Shekelle, R., *et al*., 'Dietary vitamin A and risk of cancer in the Western Electric Study', *Lancet*, 1981.)

by Richard Shekelle from Chicago in 1981 and in a large study in Japan. In all these studies, lung cancer was less common in those with a high reported intake of vitamin A, although it was suggested that the link might not be as strong with vitamin A itself as with the vitamin A related substance, beta carotene.

Studies using the case-control approach in which patients

with lung cancer were asked about their dietary patterns and were then compared to similar people without lung cancer have also been performed in the United States and Europe. In general, the association between a higher intake of carotene or retinoids and a lower rate of lung cancer has been confirmed and the stronger and more consistent link has been to carotene. Carotene is found in vegetables, as mentioned above, whereas pre-formed vitamin A is found more in fatty food. Whether there is some interaction with the fat content of the diet is not clear.

Finally, taking another approach, some seven studies have been undertaken in which cohorts of people have had blood samples taken to measure their beta carotene levels and have then been followed to find their incidence of either lung cancer or cancer in general. In general, lung cancers have occurred more in those with lower beta carotene levels, although the effect is not large.

All this evidence suggests that there is an association between vitamin A, probably in the form of carotene, and the prevention of lung cancer, and even possibly of other cancers. However, the same arguments must be applied to this evidence as we applied earlier to fat and breast cancer. That is, the association need not necessarily be a causative one. A number of alternative explanations for the association can be made. Carotene is found in fruit and vegetables, particularly carrots. People who have a diet high in fruit and vegetables will be different from other people in not only their dietary constituents but also perhaps their social background and associated behaviour. There could be some factor within these other differences which is linked in with the cancers indirectly.

This question will never be resolved by further epidemiological studies of the kind described so far. It can only be resolved by the carefully performed intervention studies of the kind that we have discussed so often. Such studies are very difficult when the dietary change is a big one like reducing the fat content or adding a large amount of fibre. They are not so difficult when they simply involve the addition of extra vitamins. For this reason, many intervention studies on the role of vitamins have been designed and developed, and some preliminary results are available. These studies are among the most important being undertaken in cancer research at the moment and, if successful, will have an immediate impact on dietary patterns for many people in the developed world. It is therefore important to look closely at what is emerging.

The first kind of intervention studies are those in which the purpose is to see if some rather indirect evidence of a role for vitamins and minerals in preventing cancer can be found. The investigators are looking to see if giving the vitamins will alter some feature of the appearance of the cells that may grow to become cancers. Therefore people with a history of heavy smoking have been examined and small samples of the lining of their airways have been looked at under the microscope. Commonly, there is evidence of a process called 'metaplasia'. This means the cells look abnormal and have some but not all of the features of cancer cells. If such people are given large doses of retinoids then some of this metaplasia will disappear. Similar changes in the lining of the mouth have been examined in people who chew betel-nut, which is a form of tobacco that can cause mouth cancer. Again, if people are given vitamin A and beta carotene the typical changes in the lining of the mouth can be reversed. Perhaps the most compelling of this kind of study has looked at the prevention of second cancers of the head and neck in patients who have already had a first cancer in that area. People who get cancers of the head and neck do so mainly as a result of exposure to smoke and alcohol. Once those cancers have been treated and cured, which they commonly can be, the cured patients are at very high risk of developing a second cancer in the head, neck or lungs which is

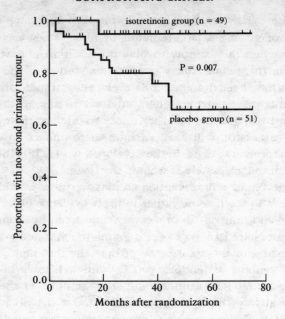

Figure 14 The protective effect of vitamin A related materials against second cancers in the head and neck.

(Prepared from data from Hong *et al.*, 'Prevention of second primary neck tumours with isotretinoin in squamous cell carcinoma of the head and neck', *New England Journal of Medicine*, 1990.)

unrelated to the first. This represents a situation in which prevention would be extremely valuable. So far, one moderately large study of this question has been reported and the results are sufficiently important to show in Figure 14. In that figure a curve is plotted to compare the development of second cancers in patients who received retinoids and in patients who did not. The difference is very large. This is very direct evidence, and the first truly direct evidence, that vitamin A related substances can prevent cancer in certain special circumstances.

Another generation of studies of this kind is now being pursued. We are aware of eleven studies of the effect of retinoids or beta carotene or vitamin E or selenium in heavy smokers, five studies of vitamins in patients with bowel abnormalities putting them at risk of colon cancer and a study of retinoids in patients with abnormalities in the neck of the womb which put them at risk of cancer of the cervix. For example, in Boston, 22,000 physicians who smoke have been allocated beta carotene supplements or a matching dummy tablet. Over the next decade they will be followed carefully to see if those who have taken beta carotene supplements have a significantly lower incidence of lung cancer than those on the dummy tablet. In Finland, a study is being sponsored by the American National Cancer Institute where 28,000 smokers are either receiving beta carotene with vitamin A or a dummy tablet. In China perhaps the most complicated study involves 20,000 Chinese who are getting vitamin A or carotene or one of seven alternative dietary supplements. They will be followed over future decades to see if they develop cancers of any site, but particularly in the gullet, which is a common site for cancer in China.

A European study, called Euroscan, is now under way. It will eventually involve 2,000 patients who have had smoking-related cancers of the head, neck or lung. They will be given beta carotene to see if this has the effect of reducing the number whom we would normally expect to develop second tumours. The Committee on Safety of Medicines gave permission in 1991 for British patients to be included in the trials.

Until the results of more prevention trials of this kind are reported we will not know the answer with any certainty. Preliminary results are quite encouraging and within the next five years or so it should be possible to give very firm advice about diet supplementation with carotene, vitamin A or its chemical relatives.

In the meantime, readers should not resort to a diet based mainly on carrots. As we have said, an excess of vitamin A causes liver damage.

Vitamin E, Vitamin C and Selenium

These are the other vitamins and minerals that have been most examined for their possible value in preventing cancer. In general, the evidence supporting their value is less than that available for vitamin A, and dietary studies are difficult to perform for vitamin E and selenium. Studies of the level of these substances in the blood of people who have subsequently been followed carefully to see if they develop cancer have been reported and are rather conflicting. At least two studies show an association between getting cancer and a low selenium level but six studies have been reported that did not show this. Similarly, for vitamin E there are two positive studies and a handful of negative studies. Overall, the evidence is still quite shaky and until clear results come in from some of the present prevention trials using vitamin E and selenium, no recommendations can be made about supplementing the diet with these substances in order to avoid cancers.

4. Chemical Additives and Cooking

There are in foods many substances which, when tested in the laboratory, can cause alteration in DNA. These include natural materials like tannins, which are found in tea, hydrazines, which are found in mushrooms, aflatoxin from mould contamination, nitrates and nitrosamines, which are found in smoked food as well as meats and fish, the organic chemicals which are produced by high-temperature cooking or heating meat, and the many environmental pollutants, pesticides and drugs used in animal husbandry. We do not know that they cause cancer in man but perhaps the most important link under investigation is between nitrates and nitrosamines, which are found in certain smoked and cooked foods, and cancer in the stomach. The most reassuring response to this suggested link is that there is a steady downward fall in the incidence of stomach cancer in the West, although it is not clear whether this is related to change in cooking and dietary habits. It would be a brave person who would suggest that we should cut tea and mushrooms out of our diets completely!

One particular feature of 'diet' which is clearly associated with cancer is the chewing of betel-nut in oriental nations. This habit consists of chewing on a quid of betel leaves, areca nuts, catechu and lime, often with tobacco added. This habit is associated with cancers of the mouth due not only to tobacco but also the other elements of the quid.

5. Obesity

'Only the effect of obesity is established beyond doubt' (Doll, 1990). There are very strong associations between obesity and certain relatively uncommon cancers but the link with common cancers is not clear, except perhaps indirectly through the fruit and vegetable content of the diet. The cancers most strongly associated with obesity are the cancers of the body of the womb in women and cancers of the gall-bladder. Studies of obesity in relation to breast cancer are still conflicting, although weak links have been claimed. Whether such links can be distinguished from the possible link to fat intake is not clear.

6. Alcohol

The link between drinking alcohol and cancer is definite but complicated. The clearest effect is on cancers of the mouth and the upper gullet and airways. This is presumably a direct effect of the alcoholic drinks as they wash over these tissues when swallowed. A most important point is that alcohol alone does not appear to have a very big effect on these cancers but that, when taken together with tobacco smoke, seems to be a powerful cause of cancer. Alcohol and tobacco smoke are responsible for the high rates of cancers in areas such as France where combined smoking and wine drinking are common.

It is possible to put some figures on this assertion for the rate of oral cancer. If we take the baseline as being a non-smoker who drinks less than one alcoholic drink each week we can give the added risk of getting an oral cancer according to how much is drunk or smoked. A non-smoker who has more than 30 alcoholic drinks a week is five or six times more likely to get oral cancer than our non-smoking, non-drinking ab-stainer. A heavy smoker who does not drink is about seven times more likely to get an oral cancer than our abstainer. However, someone who smokes more than 40 cigarettes a day and takes more than 30 alcoholic drinks per week is almost forty times more likely to get an oral cancer than the abstainer. The combined effects of alcohol and tobacco account for about three quarters of oral cancers in the Western world. Certain drinks may be particularly important. The link in France to cancer of the gullet appears to be with the home-brewed apple brandies found in the north-west of the country. Hard spirits seem to be a greater cause of cancer in the mouth than wines or beers.

Another site for cancer in which alcohol may be important is the liver. The alcohol mainly acts by causing cirrhosis of the liver, which is associated with excessive drinking for a long period. Patients with cirrhosis are very much more likely to get liver cancer than people without and to this extent alcohol underlies the cancer.

There is currently some active debate about whether alcohol

may be an important cause for two other important cancers. In some studies, an increased rate of rectal cancer is found in men who drink a lot of beer, but in other studies this has not been shown and the case is certainly not proven. For breast cancer, there has been a suggestion that the rate has increased in those who take alcohol and that women who drink a lot of alcohol are more at risk than those who drink a little. Again, the effect is not clear and there could be other factors at work.

A practical recommendation that alcohol intake should be kept at a comfortable, socially enjoyable, moderate, level is as obvious in relation to cancer as it is for other reasons. There is no evidence that complete abstention from alcohol is necessary but a heavy and prolonged intake of alcohol seems to put a person at high risk of a number of cancers.

CONCLUSIONS

The link between diet and cancer is one of the most challenging areas of current research. Some things are known with reasonable certainty, some things will be known for certain quite soon and others remain rather speculative. We believe that the link between fibre (and perhaps starch) and cancer of the large bowel is reasonably well established. The link between fat and breast cancer may not be direct and causal. Similarly, the link between fat or meat and bowel cancer may not be a direct causative one. The link between vitamin A and carotene and prevention of lung cancer and probably other cancers is still unproven, although a lot of supportive evidence exists which may be confirmed by the results of important trials in the next five years or so. Obesity is strongly associated with a number of relatively uncommon cancers. The evidence incriminating food additives and substances produced in cooking and then eaten is relatively slender except for that relating to aflatoxins from fungi, which may be important in liver cancer in the developing world. Certain nitrogen compounds in food, especially when it is smoked or preserved, are possibly implicated in stomach cancer.

So what does a practical person do about diet in order to minimize cancer risk?

These are among the most difficult recommendations we have to make because the area is so important but so uncertain. It is sensible to think about *food* rather than the nutrients of which it consists since this is the choice facing the individual. It seems also sensible to think about *enjoyable food* because only this advice is likely to be accepted. Any changes have to be *moderate*, *easy* and *cheap*. Any supplement to diet must be *simple*, *cheap* and *accessible*.

We have been impressed by some evidence and confounded by some. The science of nutrition can be rather inexact. The International Agency for Research on Cancer in Lyon has a programme to collect the dietary facts from 350,000 Europeans in the next few years. We await their results with interest and wish them good luck – they may need it.

Fruit and Vegetables

Fruit and vegetables keep coming up as beneficial in so many areas that we feel quite comfortable making a recommendation in their favour – a diet with a substantial proportion of fresh fruit and vegetables will be low in fat and meat, high in fibre and starch, high in many vitamins and in many studies is associated with low cancer risk. We cannot say which part of the fruit and vegetable diet is important. It might be the positive effect from the vitamins or fibre, or the result of taking less fat or meat. For the time being, practical advice to eat a diet with four or five portions or pieces of fresh fruit or vegetable each day seems to be supported. The studies do *not* suggest an extreme diet. It is not necessary to eat pounds and pounds of carrots – too much of several vitamins can be harmful.

Food Supplements

What about supplements? *Bran* is quite easy to increase by careful choice of a breakfast cereal as described. We recommend this even though the scientific evidence is still not complete. It is easy, palatable and harmless.

Vitamin supplements are achieving fashionable status. Do we need them? Are they safe? We advise great caution because the evidence for vitamin supplements is still incomplete and if they are taken to excess they are dangerous – particularly vitamin A. Beta carotene is safer, because only part of it is turned into the active form. Even vitamins C and D can be harmful in excess. We suggest that routine vitamin supplements are not appropriate – unless handled with caution by people at high risk. The results of studies in progress are important for this decision.

Recommendations

For our recommendations, see the box on the following page.

RECOMMENDATIONS

1. **Avoid obesity.**

2. **Eat lots of fresh fruit and vegetables of the kind you like; consider a dietary bran supplement.**

3. **Avoid a diet high in animal fat to avoid obesity, heart disease and perhaps cancer. This will happen naturally if you concentrate on fruit and vegetables.**

4. **Supplements of vitamins are still under study and probably only matter to people at high risk.**

6

Skin, Sunlight and Melanoma

Sunlight causes cancer of the skin. Fortunately, the evidence suggests that we can cope with this fact quite easily without retiring to darkened rooms for most of our lives.

In discussing this matter it is important to distinguish between two quite different types of skin cancer. The first kind is the common cancers of skin that arise from the cells which make up most of the body's covering, the epithelial cells of the skin. Although common, such skin cancers are among the most minor kinds of cancer and are usually recognized relatively easily and treated effectively by simple means. These common cancers occur in the sun-exposed areas of the body (the head, neck and hands) and tend to occur in elderly people. The second kind of skin cancer is quite different. This is known as malignant melanoma and arises from the pigmentation cells within the skin (melanocytes). These are responsible for producing the dark colour of the skin by manufacturing a material called melanin. They are distributed mainly in the deep parts of the skin, although small numbers of melanocytes are found in the eyes and in internal organs. In the body's development, melanocytes have a quite different origin from the main skin cells. Melanocytes may be collected together in the skin in the form of moles. While moles are in themselves quite innocent, they can occasionally be the focus of the development of malignant melanoma which carries with it much more serious import than other kinds of skin cancer. When a malignant melanoma develops many people can be cured simply by having the tumour excised from the skin, an operation which often leaves only a minor scar. Early detection leads to cure. However, for a proportion of patients who have melanoma, particularly those diagnosed late, the disease will persist and recur and spread to other parts of the body. It is then a serious and life-threatening condition and unlike other kinds of skin cancer.

Before going on to talk about the link between melanoma and sunlight it is worth talking a little bit about the radiations that are included in sunshine. Sunshine is made up of electromagnetic radiation of various wavelengths that include light itself. These are quite different from the radiations that we think of in association with nuclear energy or nuclear bombs, which are called ionizing radiations and are discussed in a later chapter. In sunshine the part of the electromagnetic irradiation which is of concern in relation to melanoma is called *ultraviolet irradiation* (or UV). This is divided into UVA, UVB and UVC. UVA causes the skin to darken and tan, and does not burn the skin, although too much of it can do damage at deep levels. UVB has a shorter wavelength and is therefore of greater energy. UVB ultraviolet irradiation causes redness and burning, and if you get too much UVB irradiation it causes blistering. UVC irradiation is short-wavelength, high-energy ultraviolet irradiation and is extremely damaging to skin. Fortunately, we and everything else on earth are shielded from UVC irradiation by the ozone layer – a gas layer around the earth. The ozone layer protecting us against UVC is vital to our health and that of other animals and plants. We will talk specifically about damage to the ozone layer later in this chapter. At this stage it is enough to say that there is serious concern about the damage being caused by man-made gases.

Why do we get skin cancer? The common kinds of skin cancer (called basal cell cancers or squamous cell cancers) occur as a result of exposure of susceptible skin to ultraviolet light. Pigmentation protects the skin and so it is the fair-skinned races who tend to get these common kinds of skin cancer. Once skin has become pigmented as a result of exposure to sunshine – once you have obtained your tan – then the tanned skin will give some very limited protection against burning. A tan provides the equivalent of a sun protection factor of about 2. People do not always realize that even if skin is quite tanned, sunburn is still possible. Artificial tans out of a bottle can also protect the skin slightly but are even less effective than a natural tan. They do, however, have the advantage of making it unnecessary for people to bake themselves in the sun. While we may think of a tan as attractive, a tan produced by the sun is actually a sign of skin damage.

There are other factors that can contribute to common skin cancers, including chemicals and radiation and deranged function of the body's immune system. These are rarely significant and almost all common skin cancers are directly related to sunlight. We do not understand how sunlight damages the DNA within cells of the skin to produce these common skin cancers, but we do know that individuals need a lot of exposure to sunlight to get the common skin cancers and that they are mainly a problem for fair-skinned people who have lived in the tropics and had a lot of outdoor exposure. Because they do not spread very readily and are easily removed, common skin cancers tend to be regarded by doctors as a relatively minor problem. Only occasionally will doctors have difficulties in curing this kind of skin cancer. For this reason, it is probably sufficient to adopt a relatively simple policy of watching out for new spots or blemishes on the skin and showing them to a doctor if they cause concern; this kind of skin cancer does not represent any new or developing threat to the population. We must however give more attention to melanoma, which is more complicated in its origins and more threatening in its behaviour. It represents one of the most serious trends in cancer in the latter part of this century.

Why is Melanoma Potentially So Serious?

We must first acknowledge that melanoma is not *always* serious and that early diagnosis can lead to cure by simple surgical excision. However, we cannot escape the fact that not everybody is cured in this way. In the United Kingdom 70–80 per cent of women who develop a melanoma can be cured by surgical excision of the tumour. For men the cure rate is between 50 and 60 per cent. Recurrence or spread of melanoma, when it occurs, is very dangerous because it is difficult to treat by any means. If it spreads to lymph glands near to its site of origin or if it spreads to internal organs in the body then, ultimately, it is often fatal. Early diagnosis is the key to success in the treatment of malignant melanoma. Small melanomas that are just confined to the superficial parts of the skin are almost always cured by simple surgical removal. Bigger, deeper and ulcerated melanomas are much more likely to cause problems even if an attempt is made to remove them.

The Increasing Incidence of Malignant Melanoma

The incidence of malignant melanoma is increasing rapidly in many countries. During the latter part of this century it has been doubling every ten or twelve years. The effect varies between countries and is most striking in those parts of the world where fair-skinned populations are exposed to intense sunlight. This makes Australia and the hot parts of the United States the highest-risk areas and Queensland in Australia is the melanoma 'capital' of the world. In Queensland, 30 people out of every 100,000 now get a melanoma every year. This is much higher than in Western Europe, where the figure ranges from 1.2 per 100,000 per year in Poland to over 10 per 100,000 per year in Scottish women. Within Europe, the United Kingdom overall is in the middle of the range at about 7 cases per

100,000 per year, possibly higher in Scotland, where accuracy and completeness of studies of melanoma are excellent. In many countries, the incidence is increasing rapidly, and we have illustrated this with diagrams representing the changing incidence of melanoma in the United States as reported by Dr Rige and colleagues in 1987 and in Scotland as reported by Professor MacKie and colleagues in 1992. In Scotland the current rate of increase is 7.4 per cent per year but fortunately many more melanomas are now of the thinner, less dangerous type.

Figure 15a shows the rate per 100,000 per year in dates between 1935 and the year 2000, an estimated figure. The dramatic increase is obvious. It also shows the total lifetime risk of getting a melanoma for an American citizen. This has increased from one in 1,500 in 1935 to an estimate of one in 90 in the year 2000. In view of the potential seriousness of malignant melanoma these trends have to be viewed with alarm. Upward trends in incidence have also been seen in Western Europe and in the United Kingdom. Interestingly enough, though, the public-education programmes started in 1985 in Scotland may be having an effect, for in Scotland the proportion of melanomas which fall into the thin and superficial category, and which are therefore more easily cured, has grown significantly.

The Causes of Malignant Melanoma

Determining the cause of malignant melanoma is one of the most pressing problems in cancer research today. The rapid rise of this potentially lethal cancer threatens a new epidemic. This could even be comparable to the epidemic of lung cancer which has been a feature of the twentieth century. Our understanding of the links between smoking and lung cancer is having an impact on the current trends in lung cancer and may

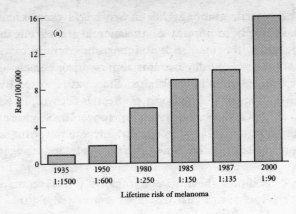

1935	1950	1980	1985	1987	2000
1:1500	1:600	1:250	1:150	1:135	1:90

Lifetime risk of melanoma

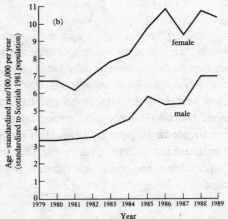

Figure 15 Risk of getting a malignant melanoma (a) in the United States (b) in Scotland.

Risk of getting a malignant melanoma in the United States has increased more than tenfold since the 1930s and is projected to rise further until the year 2000.

(Based on data taken from Balch *et al.*, 'Cutaneous melanoma', in DeVita, Hellman and Rosenberg, eds., *Cancer Principles and Practice of Oncology*, J.B. Lippincott, 1989, and Mackie *et al.*, 'Cutaneous malignant melanoma, Scotland, 1979–1989', *Lancet*, 1992.)

as we have seen, gradually be bringing this epidemic under control. It is very important that we should learn from this experience and build some such understanding into our thinking about future risks like cutaneous malignant melanoma.

We know a great deal about the causes of malignant melanoma. The most important of these is ultraviolet light in sunshine. This interacts particularly dangerously with certain kinds of skin: the risk of malignant melanoma is highest in persons with a large number of moles, poor tanning ability, a tendency to develop severe sunburn, fair or red hair, blue or green eyes and pale skin. A family history of melanoma seems to be an additional risk factor.

Sunlight

As we have indicated, melanoma is commoner in sunny climates and, in particular, in hot sunny areas occupied by fair-skinned immigrants such as Western Australia or the southwestern United States. If we take people of similar skin types, we can say that the closer they live to the equator, the more likely they are to get malignant melanoma. The risk increases when people migrate into sunnier climates. This is particularly so for children, and most studies suggest that emigrating from northern latitudes to hot sunny climes before the age of fifteen puts people at greater risk of malignant melanoma than emigrating later in life. Location of malignant melanomas on the skin does not suggest a simple relationship to sun exposure, in that melanomas are not commonest in the areas that get most sun (mainly the face and hands). In men melanomas occur most commonly on the trunk, whereas in women they occur most commonly on the leg. These are the areas that get only intermittent exposure to sunlight on the occasions when the man takes off his shirt or the girl puts on her shorts. This is probably a very important clue.

Much detailed analytical epidemiological work has been carried out to find out what particular pattern of exposure to sunlight is dangerous, and the results are now fairly conclusive. It is not total outdoor exposure to sunlight that puts people at risk of melanoma. This cancer is not associated with working outside. Indeed, careful studies have shown that malignant melanoma is less common in people who have a great deal of total outdoor sunlight exposure, or outdoor occupations, than in those who have indoor occupations and less continuous sun exposure. The pattern of sunshine exposure which is most strongly associated with cutaneous malignant melanoma is intermittent exposure of the skin among people who otherwise work indoors. Studies in Europe, Australia and North America have all shown that it is this intermittent exposure, particularly when its purpose is that of obtaining a sun tan or taking part in outdoor recreations like swimming and boating, that tends to increase the risk of melanoma. There is a very strong association of malignant melanoma with the frequency of painful sunburns in childhood.

These findings fit in very well with the distribution of melanoma in the different sexes and show a sufficiently strong link to suggest that important efforts should be made to modify behaviour in an acceptable way to reduce the risk. They suggest that the risk of the epidemic of malignant melanoma in fair-skinned people has followed from changes in our social behaviour that have prompted us to take off our clothes in public and also produced a range of incentives to get into the sun. Some of these incentives are cosmetic (tans have become fashionable), some are recreational and some result from increasing leisure time and growing opportunities for foreign travel. Most of these would be considered desirable changes and we therefore have to ask how we can retain these enjoyable activities but not run the risk of an epidemic of malignant melanoma.

Table 2
Skin Type and Sun Exposure

Type 1	White skin, never tans, always burns
Type 2	White skin, burns initially, tans with difficulty
Type 3	White skin, tans easily, burns rarely
Type 4	White skin, never burns, always tans, Mediterranean type
Type 5	Brown skin
Type 6	Black skin

Skin Type

There are many ways of considering different skin types but one useful classification is shown in Table 2.

Broadly, types 1 and 2 are those that are associated with the greatest risk of a melanoma. Types 4, 5 and 6 are pretty safe, and type 3 is probably intermediate in risk. It follows that individuals should be aware of their skin type and build this awareness into their thinking about whether it is worth their while to adopt the simple preventative measures that we will propose.

As well as the overall type of the skin, we have to consider the various freckles and moles that people get. Most of us have lots of ordinary moles, which are simple pigmented areas of little consequence. However, people with an excessive number of moles have an increased risk of malignant melanoma. Young people who have more than a hundred moles are at an increased risk. Again, possession of lots of moles should alert people to the need to take some precautions. A particular type of mole can be associated with melanoma. These are so-called 'dysplastic' moles. They are larger than usual and irregular, and tend to have variable density of colour. Possession of these can indicate a higher risk of melanoma, particularly in the presence of a family history of melanoma.

Family History

Approximately 10 per cent of cases of melanoma occur in people with a familial predisposition, and some of these will have the unusual moles called dysplastic naevi. Work on the genetics of inherited melanoma is so far incomplete, but there does seem to be a probability of a gene or chromosome which influences the risk of getting cutaneous malignant melanoma.

Other Factors

Early studies suggested the possibility of a link between malignant melanoma and the contraceptive pill, as well as a range of other factors. However, recent, well-designed and very careful studies have shown that there is no important influence of diet, alcohol, coffee, smoking, bathing habits, hair dyes, fluorescent light or the contraceptive pill on the risk of getting a melanoma. These were important possible links to explore but they are now to be discarded.

Cancer and the Ozone Layer

In the mid 1980s scientists who had studied the gases in the atmosphere made some important announcements about the ozone layer. First, the 'ozone trend' panel of scientists claimed that there had been a negative trend for the level of ozone in the atmosphere of the northern hemisphere between 1969 and 1986. Second, they drew the world's attention to the now-famous ozone hole over the Antarctic. As we have seen, the concentration of ozone in the atmosphere influences the amount of ultraviolet light that is transmitted from the sun through to the earth's surface. It has been tempting to speculate that some of the changes in the incidence of malignant melanoma may be attributable to changes in the ozone layer.

The answers to such speculation are not yet all available but a few observations can be made, particularly as a result of studies carried out in Scandinavia. Here, there has been a steady increase in the incidence of cutaneous malignant melanoma and there is also a gradient of incidence from the north to the south, with more melanoma occurring where the sun is stronger in the southern part of Scandinavia. However, the changes in ozone concentration and the changes in cutaneous malignant melanoma in Scandinavia during the 1970s and 1980s are not linked. The total amount of ultraviolet light estimated to come through the measured ozone levels has not increased greatly during the period of increasing malignant melanoma and it is much more probable that it is the behaviour of the individuals receiving the sunlight that has determined the increase. Ozone levels are undoubtedly relevant to malignant melanoma although they are not responsible for the *current* increase. None the less, some forward projections have been undertaken which suggest quite convincingly that further ozone depletion could contribute to future increases in cutaneous malignant melanomas. If behaviour patterns change and if the ozone level stabilizes, the threat can be averted. Unfortunately, there will be a time-lag before the ozone-depletion chemicals that we are producing at the present time reach the critical levels of the upper stratosphere, making any immediate stabilization of the ozone level impossible. It remains vital therefore that we should behave more responsibly.

THE PREVENTION OF MALIGNANT MELANOMA

We are sadly already some way into the early stages of an epidemic of malignant melanoma, but the means of controlling this epidemic are already to hand. They do not lie in the treatment of this cancer. Once melanoma is widespread, drugs and radiation are of very limited value. The control of the epidemic of deaths from malignant melanoma lies in its prevention and its very early diagnosis.

- *We know how to prevent malignant melanoma.*

- *We know who is most at risk.*

- *We know how to make the diagnosis easily.*

This powerful knowledge has to be handled by individuals. Governments cannot legislate or alter taxation in any way that will be particularly helpful, although they do have a role in disseminating knowledge and in reinforcing people's commitment. Malignant melanoma is a prime example of an illness which can be prevented by people taking responsible measures for themselves and their children.

For any individual, the steps in minimizing the risk of malignant melanoma are clear:

1. **Decide how far you are at risk.**

2. **Avoid intermittent intensive and unprotected exposure to sunlight.**

3. **Watch out for any of the early signs of a mole turning into a melanoma.**

1. Decide How Far You are at Risk

- *Are you white-skinned and do you sunburn easily?* If the answer to both questions is 'yes', your risk of melanoma is above average.

- *Do you have lots of moles and do you freckle easily?* Someone under forty with more than a hundred moles has an above-average risk of melanoma.

- *Do you have a family history of melanoma?* If you do, you are at increased risk of getting a melanoma yourself.

- *Do you have any unusual moles which are a bit bigger than normal or odd looking, and have you asked your doctor if they might be called dysplastic?* If you have got such moles, and particularly if your doctor says that they look dysplastic, then you are at an above-average risk of melanoma. The more of these factors that you have, the greater the attention you should pay to the second stage of preventing melanoma.

2. Control Your Sun Exposure and Your Children's

The Australians have a phrase for it: 'slip, slop, slap'. When you go out in the sun, slip on a T-shirt, slop on a hat and slap on some high-factor sun protection. This is particularly important for indoor workers who go on sunny holidays. If you want to leave some part of yourself exposed, put on a high-protection-factor sun oil. Tans can still be developed but sunburn should be avoided at all costs. If you are in a high-risk category, it would be wise to fake a tan with one of the many 'self-tanning' cosmetic preparations now on the market.

Children need to be protected. It is very rare for children to get any type of skin cancer and malignant melanoma in childhood is particularly rare. However, the sun exposure that you get in childhood may be a factor in the risk of melanoma in adult life. We therefore suggest that babies under six months should be kept out of direct sunlight. If later on they go out in the sunshine on hot summer days, a sunscreen preparation with a high protection factor is wise and it makes sense for children to wear a hat and a T-shirt and perhaps to avoid the hottest midday sun. This is particularly true on hot Mediterranean holidays.

3. Watch Your Moles

People who have moles should visit their doctor or go to a skin clinic if the mole changes

- in size
- in shape
- in colour

or if they notice inflammation, oozing, crusting, bleeding or itchiness on a mole, particularly if it is more than 7 mm (1/4 in) in diameter.

Cancer Research Campaign Checklist

The Cancer Research Campaign has produced a very useful 'Mole Watcher Leaflet'. Anyone who is in doubt should get hold of this leaflet with its useful illustrations. The checklist opposite is taken from an excellent booklet called *Question and Answer: Skin Cancer, the Sun and You* published by the Cancer Research Campaign.

Melanomas that are diagnosed easily and early when they are thin will be cured by a simple excision. This can even be done in a doctor's surgery or an out-patient clinic. The success of this approach has been shown by the outstanding work of the Scottish Melanoma Group, who have pioneered aspects of public and medical education about melanoma. This is probably directly responsible for a sustained increase in the number of thin melanomas reported and these are readily cured. Melanomas that are left until they are thick or large or widespread can often prove fatal.

Major signs

1. **An existing mole is getting larger or a new one is growing**.
   Moles do not usually grow after puberty.

2. **A mole has an irregular outline**.
   Ordinary moles are a smooth, regular shape.

3. **A mole has a mixture of different shades of brown or black**.
   Ordinary moles may be quite dark brown or black but are all one colour.

Other signs

4. **A mole is bigger than the blunt end of a pencil**.
   Most normal moles are smaller than 7 mm (1/4 in).

5. **A mole is inflamed or has a reddish edge**.
   An ordinary mole is not inflamed.

6. **A mole is bleeding, oozing or crusting**.
   Ordinary moles do not do this.

7. **A mole starts to feel different: for example, slightly itchy or painful**.
   An ordinary mole is not usually itchy or painful.

Ultraviolet Sensors

Some British scientists have been working on an ultraviolet sensor or monitor which, by using very modern technology, will be small enough and cheap enough to be convenient for personal use. Users will need to key in their skin type, the day of exposure (since people are more likely to burn in the first few days) and the protection factor of any sun cream being used. The sensor will be able to coordinate this information with its reading of the amount of ultraviolet radiation present, and the display will tell the user how much longer it is safe to stay in the sun on that occasion if sunburn is to be avoided. For those who are reluctant to change their behaviour, such a device will undoubtedly serve the useful purpose of reminding them of how little time they should spend exposed if they wish to prevent immediate sunburn (roughly, twenty minutes for an adult with skin-type 1 in the mid-June sun in the Mediterranean without any sun protection cream, increasing to about two hours with protection factor 4). However, the sensor cannot know the user's own history, whether there is a family history of melanoma or whether the user has lots of moles, and, as we have seen, migration to sunnier climes, a family history of melanoma and the presence of lots of moles can all contribute to increased risk.

Inevitably, therefore, action based on the sensor's 'advice' will be fallible. It will have its uses as a means of raising people's awareness of harmful ultraviolet radiation. In the end, though, it may give a false sense of security with regard to long-term exposure to sun and will be no substitute for common sense and action in accordance with the advice given in this chapter.

Does It Work? – the Australian Experience

We have already referred to parts of Australia as the melanoma 'capital' of the world – a dubious honour. The Australians have a special problem – many fair-skinned people, a very sunny climate and a national love of the outdoors. They have

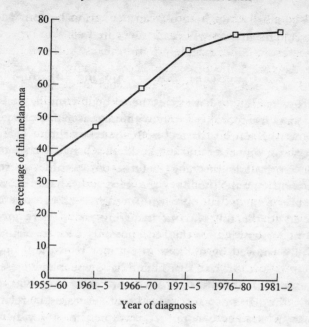

Figure 16 Thin melanomas in Australia.

(Based on data taken from Balch, C.M., and Milton, G.N., *Cutaneous Melanoma*, J.B. Lippincott, 1992, p.44, fig. 4–6.)

made great strides in tackling the problem. Australia leads the world in many areas of melanoma research and has made great contributions to our understanding of the disease. Many visitors are impressed by the level of awareness among Australians. No longer is Bondi beach a mass of exposed flesh. There is some evidence that this is beginning to pay off. The disease is still increasing but many more melanomas are being diagnosed early when they are thin and readily cured. Figure 16 shows the percentage of thin melanomas between 1955 and 1982, and the increase in the percentage of thin melanomas represents the beginning of the return from the national effort. Most of these thin melanomas can readily be cured.

The Practical Guide to Enjoying Sunshine

The advice that we have given here about avoiding malignant melanoma has to be set firmly within a reasonable perspective. Melanoma is a risk that can be eliminated by simple changes in lifestyle for ourselves and our children. Our advice should not be interpreted as meaning that the outdoor life, recreation, sport and summer holidays are necessarily harmful. Simple measures to avoid sunburn will mean that all of these can be enjoyed to the full without incurring risk. There are good reasons for wishing for this, and not only because of the great pleasure enjoyed by millions in outdoor recreations and pastimes – it is recognized that fit and happy people are less likely to get all sorts of diseases, not least cancer. We will discuss briefly the topic of exercise and work patterns in relation to cancer in another chapter. It is sufficient to say here that retaining an outdoor lifestyle and having a good time is quite compatible with a low risk of melanoma.

7

Radiation and Cancer

The term 'radiation' is associated in many people's minds with the spectre of the atomic bomb and accidents in nuclear-power generators. Images of men working in protective clothes in order to avoid lethal exposure to harmful radiation occur regularly on television and in newspapers. The Chernobyl radiation accident is still fresh in our memories and the fear of a repetition of this in densely populated parts of the Western world remains a source of public concern.

The importance of various kinds of radiation as a cause of cancer should not be underestimated, but it should not be overestimated either. First, we must deal with the matter of definition. The term 'radiation' includes very many different kinds of emission such as light, electromagnetic fields around power cables, radio waves and television waves. The relationship between ultraviolet irradiation in sunlight and skin cancer was discussed in Chapter 6 and we will touch on the relevance of electromagnetic irradiation in this chapter. However, the principal source of concern in relation to radiation involves what are known as ionizing radiations. Ionizing radiations have the characteristic of having sufficient energy to affect the chemical bonds within the materials that they hit. These chemical bonds, once broken, will cause changes that either directly or indirectly accelerate electrons from within the atoms of the target and produce reactive substances called ions – hence the name. This chemically reactive form of radiation is the principal focus of this chapter; the target materials which concern us are the large molecules like DNA, which are so biologically vital.

The most important sources of radiation are entirely natural: air, water, the food chain and minerals, and cosmic rays. Low levels of radiation come from radon gas, which is found in the soil, and a little over half of the radiation exposure of the general population probably comes from this source. There is huge variability in the exposure of people to radon depending on where they live and the construction of their homes. Cosmic rays and radiation emitted by other sources in the earth probably account for nearly one quarter of all radiation. Less than 20 per cent of irradiation is man made.

Perhaps half of the man-made radiation comes from medical X-rays and the tiny amounts of radioactivity used in medical scans. Less than 1 per cent of all the radiation of the population comes from occupational sources, nuclear fall-out or the nuclear fuel cycles.

We therefore have to modify our impression of radiation to include a steady, very low level of irradiation which is part of the normal human environment. The dose of this is difficult to estimate and will vary between different parts of the world, but is probably less than 5 milli-sieverts per year. The sievert is the unit used to measure radiation exposure in populations and we will be referring to it again. A recent estimate for the United States population was an average of 3.6 milli-sieverts per annum.

Ionizing Radiation is a Cause of Cancer

There is really no doubt that ionizing radiation can cause cancer when given under some circumstances and in sufficient doses. For this reason, radiation protection is a well-established part of our lives. Debate and controversy surround the question of how much irradiation is relevant to the causes of human cancer in the general population at the present time and what can be done about it.

The Evidence

There is an overwhelming body of evidence that large amounts of radiation will cause cancer. This has been collected throughout this century and it can be summarized as follows:

- Survivors of the atomic bombs in Hiroshima and Nagasaki have a striking excess of many cancers.

- Miners who have been exposed to excessive radon gases underground have an excess of lung cancer. Miners are also exposed to other possible factors (like asbestos) so the link with pure radon gas is still uncertain.

- Occupational exposures to radiation cause cancer; for instance, young women who ingested radium-containing paint by licking the brushes they used for painting clocks to make them luminous developed cancer.

- People treated with large doses of high-energy radiation beams are prone to develop cancer.

- Laboratory animals were treated with radiation in experiments in the early part of this century and developed an excess of cancers.

When people are exposed to large doses of radiation for a particular reason, whether it be by accident, or for military or medical purposes, it takes a long time for the cancer to develop. Ten, fifteen or twenty years may elapse, and the link may not always be easy to establish. The time taken for a cancer to develop varies between different types of cancer – leukaemia occurs a little more quickly than others (ten to twenty years) and the risk of leukaemia seems to return to normal levels after that time.

The relationship between the amount of radiation, the type of radiation and the risk of getting a radiation-induced cancer is really not very clearly worked out, particularly when low doses are concerned. It is not clear that there is a threshold below which radiation does not cause cancer. As the dose increases, the chance of inducing cancer also increases, but the nature of the relationship is not precisely understood. At very high levels of radiation, for instance, the chances of inducing a cancer may actually decrease, perhaps because most of the target cells are in fact killed outright. Some human tissues are more susceptible to radiation-induced cancer than others. The bone marrow seems to be the most vulnerable, and adult leukaemia is therefore one of the most important radiation-induced cancers. The breast and thyroid gland are also very sensitive to radiation.

Prevention of Radiation-induced Cancer

Since we know ionizing radiation can cause cancer we must minimize the risk to the general population and concentrate particularly on those for whom there is special concern, such as workers in the radiation industry. In general, the science of radiation protection is now well developed. The historical examples of occupational exposure, like the painters of watch faces mentioned above, serve as chilling warnings of the consequences of relaxing radiation protection, but in general most workers in the radiation industry are working at levels of exposure which are associated with only negligible increases in cancer risk. There is no cause for complacency and even more strict radiation protection regulations are now being imposed. The new regulations in the United Kingdom for substances hazardous to health will help to document, strengthen and enforce the regulations.

The risk of nuclear accident or the deliberate use of nuclear radiation in warfare remains with us. Minimizing this risk is perhaps one of the most crucial roles of government in cancer prevention.

If exposure to large doses of irradiation, in occupations or accidents or warfare, are now avoidable, the focus of radiation protection comes down to the low doses of irradiation which are present in everyday life.

At present, little can be done about the exposure to natural irradiation in the environment. It probably contributes a relatively small amount to the total cancer risk and certainly is very much less important than major factors like smoking or diet. Medical exposure to ionizing radiation in diagnostic X-rays should be kept to a minimum. New techniques and new machines are aimed at minimizing dose levels and reducing the amount of tissue X-rayed. It is pretty clear that, within these technical limitations, the benefits of irradiation are much greater than the risk of increased cancer, if any, at such low doses.

People should not, however, have X-rays too frequently. Dental X-rays should not be given to people with normal and healthy teeth and gums more often than once every two years. It is important to wear a special apron when having a dental X-ray and your dentist will provide this for you. It is particularly important to avoid the irradiation of the unborn child and babies in the first year of life. All doctors are concerned to minimize the use of X-rays in pregnancy and in early life, and X-rays should only be used when there is a very clear need for the information that they generate.

Examples of Radiation Hazards

Two examples of the link between radiation and cancer have attracted recent public attention. The first of these has been the question of an increased risk of cancer in servicemen who attended the United Kingdom Atmospheric Nuclear Test Programme at Christmas Island in 1958 and the second is the possibility of an increased risk of cancer in the children of workers in the nuclear-power industry. A third risk, much less discussed publicly, arises from radon gas in soil.

Testing Nuclear Bombs

In the 1950s, the United Kingdom tested its nuclear arsenal in atmospheric tests based on or around Christmas Island. Throughout late 1957 and much of 1958 a series of tests was performed. The details of these are still subject to official restriction but a great deal has been revealed. Some of the bombs were air dropped and burst over the ocean, some were balloon suspended, some burst over sea and some exploded above the island. Some were in the kilo-ton and some in the low megaton yield of radiation. Most of these explosions were many times the power of the bombs dropped on Hiroshima and Nagasaki.

Some 22,347 UK nationals, mainly servicemen, were present during one or more nuclear-weapon tests at Christmas Island. We know surprisingly little about how much exposure to irradiation there was. The vast majority of men did not carry radiation dosimeters and these only detect external irradiation anyway. The men who were subsequently monitored were not even very representative of the group as a whole, because the people who carried monitors were mainly the specialized scientific staff and not the servicemen. We do know that the personal film badges that were worn by the staff who were monitored would not have recorded exposure to radioactive materials that were inhaled or swallowed or to neutrons, a particular kind of ionizing irradiation. However, the evidence is fairly good that the amount of radiation to which the servicemen were exposed was, in the main, quite small. If the annual exposure to irradiation in the Western world in the general population is less than 5 milli-sieverts it should be particularly interesting to know how many servicemen had more than this during their time at

Christmas Island. Among the 1,373 who carried monitors, only 483 individuals received 5 milli-sieverts or more. Eighty participants at the test were recorded as receiving 50 milli-sieverts or more and most of these eighty individuals were the crew of aircraft which sampled radioactive clouds after the explosions. We can now see that this aspect of the testing exercise was very ignorant and foolish.

The overall mortality in the servicemen who went to Christmas Island and a comparable group of servicemen of similar age has been found to be very similar, both for cancer and other causes. In both groups, the early mortality was rather less than would have been expected in the general population, reflecting the fact that these were relatively fit young men. However, even though more than thirty years have now elapsed, no *overall* excess of cancer has been found among the men who were present at Christmas Island. This is the finding of a very long follow-up study of all participants in UK atmospheric nuclear tests carried out by the National Radiation Protection Board. The results are not however completely comforting. The study has shown that the participants in the tests have experienced a significant excess of leukaemia. The servicemen who attended the nuclear tests were tracked down and their medical records were compared to those of a similar group of servicemen who had not attended the tests. The mortality from leukaemia and another bone-marrow cancer called multiple myeloma was much higher in the nuclear-test servicemen than in the comparison group. Among the few other differences found, perhaps the most interesting was that the incidence of lung cancer was lower in the Christmas Island group than in those who stayed at home. Perhaps they were sufficiently concerned about their experience to stop smoking!

Does this mean that the leukaemia and the myeloma occurred as a result of attending the nuclear tests? We think they probably did. It is difficult to prove this with certainty. There were some inconsistencies in the findings. In particular, there seems to have been an unusually low rate of myeloma in the group of servicemen who did not go to Christmas Island compared with that of the general population of England and Wales. However, we do know that leukaemia and multiple myeloma are among the cancers most likely to be induced by radiation. Some additional evidence comes from other reports of an excess of leukaemia in people who attended nuclear tests in Utah in the United States but these studies are not completely convincing. Scientifically the case is unproven but the balance of probabilities suggests that very low doses of irradiation exposure in the servicemen were responsible for an increase in the risk of leukaemia and myeloma. The impact of this on the group overall was relatively small although, of course, the impact on the individuals concerned (between fifteen and twenty in the British tests) was very great. The example serves to illustrate the need for constant vigilance in the process of avoiding radiation-induced cancers and argues, if any additional argument is necessary, against any further atmospheric tests of nuclear devices.

The Children of Nuclear-power Workers

For many years it has been known that there is a certain clustering of childhood leukaemia around nuclear-power installations. Scientists continue to bend their minds to the problem of explaining these observations. The first and most obvious explanation would be that the children are in some way exposed to radiation. In fact, the radiation exposure is probably only of a very low level and it does not seem to be the cause. In the late 1980s, scientists from the University of Southampton pointed out that some of the leukaemia cases occurred in families of workers in the nuclear installations. They suggested the possibility that the cause of leukaemia in the children of such workers might lie in damage occurring as a result of radiation exposure which altered the genetic material of the fathers' sperm. This serious and anxiety-provoking possibility remains a subject of careful scientific investigation. Until the matter is resolved it reinforces the need for stringent control of radiation exposure in the workplace.

Electromagnetic Fields

Electrical sources like power cables emit alternating electromagnetic fields at very low frequencies. For many years there was no special concern that these might be associated with cancer. However, in 1979 an epidemiological study was published by Drs Wertheimer and Leeper suggesting that children who lived within a short distance of alternating electromagnetic fields were at increased risk of some cancers. This observation has generated a vast amount of discussion, research and investment in research into the possible harmful effects of electromagnetic fields. The work is incomplete and it is hard to draw conclusions. Indeed, our colleague Professor Ray Cartwright, in an article in the *British Journal of Cancer*, concluded 'it is not surprising that some confusion exists in the minds of the scientific community and the general public as to the reality of these risks'.

Briefly, most of the scientific evidence, although not yet conclusive, suggests that the risk, if it exists, is small. The energy emitted by these low-frequency electrical sources is at the low end of the electromagnetic (EM) spectrum, much below that of radio waves or ultraviolet rays. Electromagnetic fields are not ionizing and do not even produce heat. There has not been much work in the laboratory, but such work as has been done does not show any consistent evidence of cancer causation by electromagnetic irradiation from electrical sources. Wertheimer and Leeper produced the only evidence which causes concern. They looked at the incidence of childhood leukaemia in relation to electromagnetic fields and said that it was higher in children who had a high exposure to EM fields. Since then, studies have looked at occupations where there is believed to be an excess of exposure to electrically generated electromagnetic irradiation. Such occupations include those of linesmen, power-station workers, telecommunication workers, electrical engineers, nuclear-shipyard electricians, radio and television repairers and assembly-line workers. On balance, the studies suggest there may be a small excess risk of leukaemia in these workers but it is difficult to link this conclusively to electromagnetic irradiation. There is no good, conclusive evidence that they are actually exposed to more electromagnetic irradiation than the general population and it is quite possible that they are exposed to other leukaemagens (leukaemia-inducing agents) such as chemicals in the workplace. Studies which have attempted to reproduce the observations of a link between childhood leukaemia and overhead power cables have, in general, been unconvincing but are continuing. The results of these investigations are very difficult to interpret because the studies are small and the documentation of the actual exposure to electromagnetic irradiation as a result of the power lines is rather imprecise.

Those currently investigating this problem in North America and Europe will try even harder to tease out the answers. This will take years, and will cost the power industry and government large sums of money. There will be much more speculation but, at present, the scientific evidence seems to point to the following conclusion drawn by Ray Cartwright in his recent article: 'We are thus looking forward to many more years of speculation surrounding the supposed adverse health effects of electromagnetic fields at very low frequencies with respect to leukaemia, despite the fact that our present scientific knowledge points at the very best to a minute risk of electromagnetic fields verging on the point of non-existence.'

Radon in the Soil

In uranium mines, the gas radon and some of its radioactive products accumulate in the air, together with other gases and dust. This has been identified as a cancer risk for many years even though it remains unproven that the radon gas is *by itself* the cause of the cancers. The quantities of radioactive radon gas in the air, even in uranium mines, are very small and, traditionally, have been defined in a unit known as 'the working level month'. A miner who is exposed to four working level months has a 60 per cent increased risk of lung cancer and, if he is a smoker, this means a very high risk indeed. Up to 8 per cent of miners working in uranium mines develop lung cancer as a result of exposure to radon gas and other products. The more radon gas they are exposed to the more likely they are to get lung cancer, and it is possible to calculate the relationship between the dose of radon and the risk of lung cancer quite accurately.

Precautions and screening and reduced exposure in the workplace are now standard occupational safety measures for uranium miners in the United States.

The interest in radon gas has now shifted to questions about exposure of the general population outside the workplace. Radon gas comes from the rocks and soil and accumulates in houses where there is limited ventilation. Radon actually accounts for a very large proportion of human irradiation, far in excess of cosmic rays and other naturally occurring radioactive substances. The background irradiation in the environment is something like 1 milli-sievert (this unit was discussed above, where we said that the general population should not receive more than 5 milli-sieverts in a year). The 1 milli-sievert that people get in the general environment does not vary much. In contrast, the amount of radioactivity due to radon gas in houses varies tremendously. In the United Kingdom, the average concentration in a house leads to about 1 milli-sievert per year of irradiation. However, in otherwise ordinary houses this concentration can vary from $\frac{1}{10}$ milli-sievert to 1,000 milli-sieverts! Most of the general population is exposed to only small levels of irradiation from radon gas but these might contribute significantly to the number of lung cancers. One epidemiological study suggested that as many as 25 per cent of lung cancers in non-smokers arise as a result of exposure to radon and its related radioactive material. Further studies are necessary, particularly because the exposure to radon in houses (as a gas) is different from that in mines (as fine particles of rock and with other possibly relevant materials).

The International Commission on Radiological Protection has tried to set some standards for ideal radon exposures. The upper accepted level is set by a calculation that says that no one should be exposed to a quantity of radon that would more than double their lifetime risk of lung cancer. Studies conducted in the United States and Sweden suggest that the risk of lung cancer is indeed higher in people who live in dwellings on top of soil and rocks which have an increased risk of yielding radon, and we cannot afford to ignore these findings.

If the link between radon and cancer is confirmed, the solution to the risk of radon gas lies in the measurement of radon concentrations in individual houses and in increasing the ventilation of those that have higher-than-acceptable levels. In the United Kingdom, the surveying of houses is under active consideration and may be implemented in the coming decade. In the meantime, individuals in parts of the UK who are worried about reports of high radon levels in houses in their locality can apply to the National Radiation Protection Board for a free test reading.

CONCLUSIONS

For protection against ionizing radiation-induced cancers we have to rely heavily upon government and its agencies and health-care workers. There is not much room for action by the individual. This is in contrast to the possibilities of prevention of melanoma by individuals who are exposed to ultraviolet light, a special form of irradiation distinct from ionizing radiations. Pressure on governments should be maintained if we are to keep the risks of radiation-induced cancer at a low level.

New measures have recently been proposed in the UK by the National Radiation Protection Board. First, they looked at exposure to X-rays in hospital tests and found it to be unnecessarily high in some cases. More stringent and precise limits are being introduced. In the environment, the level of contamination by nuclear installations is low but might still be further improved. The board recommended a reduction by 40 per cent to 0.3 milli-sieverts a year.

Careful surveillance of radiation exposure must remain a high priority.

8

Sex, Hormones and Reproduction

Sex, hormones and reproduction play a major part in the lives of men and women, and it is not surprising that each has some features which are related to cancer risk and which provide some potential for cancer prevention. The cancers that are of greatest importance are those which arise in tissues that are sensitive to sex hormones – the breast and womb in women and the prostate gland in men. Most other tissues in the body are influenced to some extent by a wide range of hormones but these are the parts of the body where hormones have the biggest impact and are therefore most implicated as a cause of cancer.

Sexual activity, as well as being a matter of reproduction and hormones, can also of course be involved in the transfer of infectious agents. Most recently this has become well publicized because of the AIDS epidemic, but we need to examine carefully other less obvious and dramatic possibilities that may link sexual activity to certain kinds of cancer.

Because sex and reproduction are so important to us, suggestions of cancer risks that are related to sex, hormones and reproduction are often those which attract the closest attention. In this chapter we shall dispel myths and draw attention only to those factors for which there is some real evidence of a link with cancer, and which therefore have the potential for prevention.

BREAST CANCER

Factors Associated with Breast Cancer

Breast cancer does not occur in children and the first cases are seen in the late teens and in the early twenties. At that age, the disease is rare but its frequency increases rapidly up to age fifty and then continues to increase, but less rapidly, thereafter. As we noted in the chapter on diet, there is a great deal of variation in breast cancer risk between countries. Social class is also a factor and the breast cancer rate at any age is usually considerably greater in higher socio-economic classes than in lower socio-economic classes. Whether this difference relates to diet or to other factors is still not clear.

The breast is highly sensitive to hormones, particularly oestrogens. Breasts develop with the hormonal changes in puberty in girls. The cyclical changes in hormones in the menstrual cycle affect breast tissues and their effect can sometimes be the cause of considerable discomfort. Hormones in pregnancy cause the breasts to increase in size and after delivery it is hormones that cause milk production. The most direct link between breast cancer and female hormones is very obvious – breast cancer is very rare in men.

An important relationship between hormones and breast cancer is that the careful use of hormones can be a valuable aid to the treatment of breast cancer. Such therapy used to be carried out with the naturally occurring female hormones, oestrogens and progesterones, and these are still used. However, the best available drug at present is not a naturally occurring hormone but a synthetic drug called Tamoxifen. This is remarkably well tolerated and is a very useful treatment for established cancers. Although we do not know exactly how Tamoxifen works, we know that it partly blocks naturally occurring hormones which can stimulate the growth of breast cancer.

The features of the reproductive and hormonal cycles in women which are associated with an increased risk of breast cancer are:

- *An early onset of menstruation.* Women whose periods begin at the age of twelve or before and who rapidly establish regular cycles are several times more likely to develop breast cancer than those whose menstruation does not start until after the age of thirteen.

- *A late menopause.* Women whose menopause occurs before the age of forty-five have only about half the risk of breast cancer of those whose menopause occurs after the age of fifty-five.

- *No pregnancies, or late pregnancies.* Women who have lots of babies are less likely to get breast cancer than women who do not. This explains why breast cancer is commoner in single women and in married women who have no children. Most of this effect is determined by the age of the mother when the first baby is born. Women who have their first baby under the age of twenty have only about half the risk of breast cancer of a woman who never has a child. If the first child is born at around about thirty to thirty-five years then there is virtually no protective effect and the risk of getting breast cancer is about the same as that of a woman who has never had a child. If the first child is born when the mother is more than thirty-five years old then the risk of getting breast cancer is probably slightly greater than that of the childless women.

No one can extend these observations into a recommendation that women should all have their children early. There are many other factors that operate in these decisions. Nevertheless, the observations seem to be real and cannot be ignored. They lead us to reinforce the advice that women aged fifty to sixty-four should have careful breast cancer screening. Such advice would be particularly true for those whose age at first motherhood was more than thirty.

Hormones, Breast Cancer and Prostatic Cancer

The female hormone, oestrogen, is an important influence on the growth of the breast and testosterone, the male hormone, is an important influence on the growth of the prostate. There is a wealth of evidence, unsurprisingly, that the cancers derived from these tissues can be sensitive to these hormones. The relationship is not a simple, straightforward one. As we have mentioned, very high concentrations of sex hormones can actually be used for treating breast cancer, as can drugs derived from the sex hormones, like Tamoxifen. Removing the hormonal drive can also be a valuable treatment and this can be achieved with drugs for men with prostatic cancer. Another useful treatment can be achieved by switching the hormone drive. If oestrogens, the female hormones, are given to men with prostatic cancer, the prostatic cancer will often improve. The oestrogens serve to counteract the effect of the male sex hormones. We do not know all of the factors that influence the interaction of sex hormones and these common cancers, but we do know that the relationships are important.

The Contraceptive Pill and Breast Cancer

In the early 1960s oral contraceptive pills were introduced in the United States and Western Europe. Their use spread rapidly during the 1970s and early 1980s but has now declined. In the early years, the Pill was used to help plan the families of older women. Many careful studies were carried out to see if there were any effects of the Pill on breast cancer risk, and for all groups in this older age group the results were reassuring.

No study has ever suggested that there is an increased risk of breast cancer from the use of oral contraceptives by those in their late twenties or thirties, perhaps the commonest married reproductive years.

During the 1970s, the pattern of Pill usage changed and it was more widely used by younger women in their late teens and early twenties. This use of the Pill was associated with changes in social attitudes and behaviour which involved earlier sexual activity and increased sexual activity outside marriage. Studies of the younger women who used the Pill are not quite so reassuring. A group of research workers led by Malcolm Pike suggested in the early 1980s that oral contraceptives that had been used before a first pregnancy, or before the age of twenty-five were associated with a small but significant increased risk of breast cancer. Since that time, a series of case-control studies have been carried out which have included such young patients. The results of some thirteen case-control studies have been published, including those from a large national study in the UK of over 750 cases of breast cancer. A very large study was also carried out in the United States (the so-called Cancer and Steroid Hormone Study published in 1985 by Stadel and colleagues) in which there were over two thousand cases. Epidemiologists still argue about the relative merits of these studies, and the possibilities of bias have been described in almost every case. However, on balance, the studies do seem to show a small increase in the relative risk of getting breast cancer if the Pill was used in these early phases of the reproductive life in women. No study suggests that the Pill protects against breast cancer. We believe that we should accept that there is a small increased risk of breast cancer associated with oral contraceptive use at an early age. This small increase in risk is confined to those who used oral contraceptives during their late teens and early twenties and does not relate to women who used the Pill later in life. It also relates only to those who have got breast cancer relatively early (up to age forty); this is simply because insufficient time has elapsed to know what the risk will be later in life for those who took the Pill very early.

At present, the impact of the Pill on the overall risk of breast cancer in the population is very small. This is because breast cancer before the age of forty is still a rare disease. The chances of getting breast cancer before the age of forty in the United Kingdom are about 1 in 500. If we accept that the case-control studies do indeed suggest that there is an increased risk for breast cancer for those who took the Pill before the age of twenty-five, then the risk for these women of getting breast cancer before they reach the age of forty is still only about 1 in 300. What we do not yet know is what their lifetime risk of getting breast cancer may be. The overall lifetime risk for a woman in the United Kingdom is 1 in 14. If the effect which we have already seen for those who took the Pill earlier in life lasts throughout their lives, then the risk could be increased to 1 in 6 or 1 in 8 and would be a very real cause for concern. There is no evidence that this is yet happening but it is an important reason for very careful monitoring of breast cancer risks in all age groups in all countries where the Pill was widely used during the 1970s and 1980s in young women.

On the other hand, we should not ignore the well-established benefits of the Pill. It is clearly protective against ovarian cancer and reduces the risk by 50 per cent.

Hormone Replacement Therapy (HRT) and Cancer

The effects of the menopause on the health of a woman are well recognized. The immediate symptoms may be flushing, emotional upsets and change in sex drive. The physical changes in the body's structure are also well recognized. It is clear, too, that there is a link between the menopause and osteoporosis, the thinning of the bones which can result in loss of height in the spine and the forward bending which is so typical in very elderly women. Osteoporosis also places women at risk of fracturing their hips, which is a serious condition in its own right and which is potentially very dangerous if it occurs in an elderly person with poor general health. The menopause therefore has a very real medical 'down side'.

Many of the problems of the post-menopausal age for a woman can be avoided by hormone replacement. When menopause occurs the ovaries stop making the oestrogens and progesterones which cause the menstrual cycle and maintain physical well-being and the strength of bones. If they can be replaced by tablets or skin patches then many of the health hazards or problems should be avoided. For example, the loss of sex drive and general body tone can be restored by hormone replacement therapy after the menopause. Osteoporosis can be avoided. It also now seems highly likely that the risk of heart disease (common in men and less common in women) can be reduced in women later in life by maintaining their female hormone levels. This is important because heart attacks are a significant cause of death in older women, even more common than breast cancer.

We have already said that the sex hormones in women can play a part in the development of cancers of the breast and of the lining of the womb. It is therefore appropriate to ask whether hormone replacement therapy will lead to a higher risk of breast cancer.

Part of the answer is now clear. The replacement of female hormones *by oestrogen alone* in the post-menopausal period is associated with a small increased risk of breast cancer. The risk is about 1.3 to 1.9 times that of someone who does not use hormone replacement therapy. It is most marked in those who use only oestrogen and who use the oestrogen in high doses. High doses for a long time carry a significant risk of breast cancer. Oestrogen, given by itself, is also associated with an increased risk of cancer of the lining of the womb. However, the risks of using low doses of oestrogen are very small.

Another important development has been the use of hormone replacement therapy using a mixture of the two female hormones, oestrogens and progesterones. The effect on breast cancer risk of adding progesterone to hormone replacement therapy is not yet fully evaluated because this change has taken place only in the last ten years or so. The studies that are so far available almost all suggest that oestrogen–progesterone replacement therapy is not associated with any increased risk of breast cancer. We shall have to wait longer before we can be entirely confident about this because the studies have been short, small and not as water-tight in their scientific method as those carried out earlier. We can be very cautiously optimistic that the breast cancer risk associated with hormone replacement therapy may be minimized or avoided altogether by careful choice of hormones.

Where does the balance lie? Hormone replacement therapy can make women feel better, reduce their risk of fractures and deformities of the spine and probably reduce their risk of heart attack. On the other hand there remains concern about the possibility of a small increase of breast cancer. At present we feel the balance probably favours the very careful use of hormone replacement therapy for women who fully understand the risks and the benefits and the need for very careful monitoring. It would certainly be wise for any doctor recommending HRT to ensure that the woman has had a clear mammogram before starting the therapy and will be included in the screening programmes discussed later in the book.

Hormones to Prevent Breast Cancer

Hormones can be a factor in the cause of breast cancer but, as we have already indicated, the risks associated with hormones can be kept to a minimum if we are careful about how we use them. We also know they can be used in the treatment of breast cancer. What about its prevention? The answers here are not clear but the potential is very considerable. Tamoxifen is a very simple and effective drug and its long-term use for the treatment of breast cancer is not associated with much toxicity. In other words, it does not poison as it cures. Could it be given to large numbers of women who are at risk of breast cancer in order to prevent the disease? The answer is unknown but is probably one of the most exciting questions in the management of breast cancer at present. As a preventative measure, it would be simple and therefore readily accepted by a large number of people. As we said when discussing the sort of dietary measures that can realistically be introduced for prevention of cancer, we cannot expect to change people's lives completely, although we might expect small interventions to be acceptable.

We cannot offer Tamoxifen to every woman. The risk of breast cancer is one in 14 in a lifetime and therefore 13 women would be taking it for no purpose. Can we choose who should be offered this approach? At present, it can be said that there are populations at high risk of breast cancer. These are defined by a very strong family history (a mother or sister with the disease), a previous breast cancer in the other breast or the presence of certain abnormalities in the breast seen on X-ray. Careful choice of people to be offered Tamoxifen as a preventative agent could therefore be carried out on the basis of these known risk factors. In the United Kingdom at present, a study to measure the benefits and risks of this approach is planned. In the United States, such a study got under way in 1992. In between five and ten years' time we will know whether Tamoxifen prevention will be another way in which we can have a major impact upon the development of breast cancer in women with a higher-than-average risk.

CARCINOMA OF THE LINING OF THE WOMB

Carcinoma of the endometrium or lining of the womb is the commonest of the cancers arising from the female reproductive tract. It tends to have slightly less emphasis in the medical literature and in popular awareness than the other two common cancers – those of the ovary and of the cervix. This is because it has a low death rate and this, in turn, is primarily because it is usually diagnosed when the cancer is early, confined to the uterus and easily removed by surgery.

It occurs between the ages of fifty-five and sixty, and bears a close relationship to the hormone pattern of the woman. A late menopause or the administration of high doses of oestrogen for a long time as part of hormone replacement therapy are powerful risk factors for endometrial cancer. When hormone replacement therapy is given by a mixture of oestrogen and progesterone there does not appear to be any increased risk of endometrial cancer and the risk may well be diminished. This observed difference is probably the strongest evidence available at present for the use of mixed hormone replacement therapy and is certainly much clearer than that for cancer of the breast.

CANCER OF THE CERVIX

Sexual Activity and Cancer of the Cervix

The neck of the womb or cervix is an important site of cancer in women. It differs from cancer arising in the lining of the body of the womb in a number of important ways. It occurs at an earlier age, usually between forty-five and fifty-five. Abnormalities can be seen in the neck of the womb many years before a cancer develops. This is the basis of the cervical smear screening test discussed in Chapter 13, and these abnormalities are probably the best-known example of a pre-malignant change for a common cancer. The abnormalities are shown by changes in the cells which cover the neck of the womb – the epithelium. These cells change their shape and general appearance and their relationship to each other gradually, and these changes are limited to the epithelium. Only when they break out from the epithelium into the underlying tissues of the neck of the womb is invasive cancer diagnosed. Finding these cells in smears of cells taken from the neck of the womb is the basis of the important screening tests which will, if carefully and accurately applied, reduce the risks of cervical cancer very significantly in future.

Cancer of the cervix is the cancer which is most clearly linked to sexual activity. It is more frequent in women who begin sexual intercourse early, women who have larger numbers of sexual partners, women who become pregnant early, women who have many children and among prostitutes. The converse is true; cancer of the cervix is infrequent in women who have no children or have inactive sex lives (such as nuns) and in women who marry once and have no children. It is also quite infrequent in Jewish and Muslim women and it has been suggested that circumcision in their partners is an important preventative factor. This has not been proved.

How does sexual activity lead to cancer of the cervix? It seems quite likely that it occurs as a result of transfer of an infectious agent. Two viruses are the leading candidates. Herpes simplex virus infection is commoner in women who have cancer of the cervix than in the general population. The virus can be transferred by sexual intercourse and can produce a venereal disease which occurs as an unpleasant, short-lived illness. It is, however, particularly troublesome because it tends to recur. Although herpes viruses can be found in patients who have cancer of the cervix, the evidence that they actually cause the cancer is far from clear. The viruses may just be 'passengers' that one would expect to find transferred by venereal contact in the same population as those who get cancer of the cervix as a result of their sexual history. The other virus is one of the human papilloma virus family. These are the viruses that cause warts on the skin but there are many different types. Two particular human papilloma viruses are found in patients with cancer of the cervix. The evidence that they cause the disease is still not conclusive but it is a little stronger than that for herpes simplex viruses. The evidence is derived from the frequency of the association between papilloma viruses and cancer of the cervix, and from biological studies of the cells of cervical cancer. Human papilloma viruses are found in these cells both in the form of whole viruses and parts of viruses. Evidence is accumulating that the papilloma virus is an important factor in cancer of the cervix but is, as we have said, not yet conclusive.

CANCER, AIDS AND SEXUAL CONTACT

The link between sexual contact and AIDS has been well publicized. The details of this link are beyond the scope of this book but we do feel that we should at least comment on the association between AIDS and cancer. There is such an association. Patients who have AIDS are at greater risk of cancer than those who do not have AIDS. The cancers that occur are in general those that are associated with an alteration in the body's immune function. The primary problem with AIDS is this alteration in immune function, and AIDS patients are very vulnerable to infections. The altered immune function also makes them vulnerable to certain cancers. Kaposi's sarcoma is rare in the general population and occurs mainly in the skin. This unusual kind of cancer is much commoner in AIDS patients and occurs both on the skin and in the lining of the gut. Lymphomas are cancers of the immune system and they occur more frequently in AIDS patients. Other cancers that are associated with virus infection, like cancers of the liver and cancers of the neck of the womb, are in fact somewhat more frequent in populations with a high risk of AIDS infection. The links, if any, have not been fully worked out and some of the observations have been limited to seeing if there are changes in the frequency of some cancers among young unmarried men. Young unmarried men will include those populations most at risk of AIDS – in particular male homosexuals who do not practise safe sex – but will also include heterosexuals and homosexuals who do practise safe sex; we must therefore treat cautiously observations based on this group.

The preventative measures to be taken in relation to cancers associated with AIDS are the same as those for AIDS itself. The practice of safe sex and the avoidance of multiple sexual partners can minimize the risk of AIDS. Transfer of human immune deficiency virus (HIV) in blood products, such as tragically occurred earlier with haemophiliacs, will not be repeated and it does seem at the time of writing that some of the most ominous predictions for the spread of AIDS in the heterosexual populations of Western countries are not being fulfilled. The threat has not passed, however, and the practice of safe sex and the limiting of numbers of sexual partners for the heterosexual population as well as the homosexual population are crucial to minimizing the AIDS risk and avoiding the increased risk of cancer that comes with this disease.

CONCLUSIONS

Sexual activity, reproduction and the hormonal environment in the body are all potent forces influencing the risk of cancer. They certainly generate important opportunities for prevention. Taking account of the reproductive pattern as it relates to breast cancer makes a lot of sense, and the prevention of breast cancer by treatment with carefully selected hormone-related substances like Tamoxifen may be a powerful way of avoiding breast cancer in future. Careful modification and implementation of hormone replacement therapy and monitoring of patients who use oral contraceptive pills are also advisable. Modifications to sexual practice which limit the number of sexual partners and increase the practice of safe sex should have an impact on AIDS and cancer of the cervix. Condoms can not only help to prevent AIDS and to cut down the risk of cervical cancer but also minimize the risk of other sexually transmitted diseases and serve as an excellent contraceptive device. Screening for cancer of the cervix should be effective if it is properly organized. There is some cause for cautious optimism on this front in future decades.

9

Cancer, the Workplace and Environmental Pollution

THE WORKPLACE

Most adults spend half their waking hours at work and some may spend much more than this. Many workplaces give rise to particular concerns and in this chapter we will look at some examples. In addition, it is reasonable to ask whether changing patterns of occupation are likely to influence the incidence of cancer.

The list of associations that have been established between workplace exposure and subsequent cancer is long. However, the number of examples where there is need for new measures or new action on the part of individuals in order to reduce the cancer risk is relatively small. The best-documented associations are given in the table.

This list is not comprehensive but demonstrates that some very specific associations have been shown to exist in particular industries and have now largely been dealt with by the introduction of careful controls in the Western world. Sadly, such controls are not worldwide. There is growing concern as our knowledge increases of the patterns of cancer in Eastern Europe, where environmental exposure to cancer-causing agents in the workplace has been much less well controlled than in Western Europe and the United States.

Table 3
Cancer in the Workplace

Workplace exposure	Industry	Cancer caused	Measures required
Radioactivity	Nuclear power	Many, particularly leukaemia	Radiation protection to minimize exposure to radiation
Asbestos	Building	Mesothelioma (chest-wall cancer)	Replacement of asbestos in construction
Organic chemicals	Dyeing and engineering	Bladder cancer	Control of substances hazardous to health (COSHH) in the workplace
Unknown	Farming	Multiple myeloma (bone-marrow cancer)	Unknown
Arsenic	Mining, smelting and pesticide manufacture	Lung, skin and liver	COSHH
Wood dust	Furniture manufacturing	Nasal sinuses	Air filtration and masking
Vinyl chloride	Manufacturing of polyvinyl chloride	Angiosarcoma of the liver	COSHH
Nickel, mustard gas, chromium	Various industries	Lung	COSHH
Benzene	Leather industry	Leukaemia	COSHH

Asbestos and Mesothelioma: the Solution of a Problem Yet to Come

Many features of the difficulty of dealing with cancers induced by environmental pollutants can be demonstrated by looking carefully at the relationship between asbestos and cancer. Asbestos has been widely used for many decades because of its strength and resistance to fire. Various forms of the material are used in insulation, cement production, pottery manufacture, flooring, brake linings, roofing, packing and textiles. Asbestos is found in cement deposits and piping systems.

Widespread use of asbestos developed during the nineteenth century. Towards the turn of the century the first identification of a medical hazard from asbestos exposure was made. It was reported that in both English and French asbestos textile mills workers developed lung scarring ten or fifteen years after beginning work in the factories, and that this often led to death from lung damage. By the 1920s doctors were describing the lung damage as being directly due to exposure to asbestos and the term 'asbestosis' came into use in the United Kingdom in the 1930s. The amount of asbestos exposure was restricted by law and many felt that the problem had been solved.

Unfortunately, the problem was not solved. During the 1940s and 1950s suspicions about a link between asbestos and lung cancer emerged, and in 1955 Richard Doll reported in a case-control study that there was a strong association between asbestos and lung cancer. In the 1950s and 1960s it became clear that the association of asbestos was not only to cancer of the lung but also to a malignant process known as mesothelioma in which the cancer arises in the lining of the chest and, less frequently, the lining of the abdomen. This disease was first reported clearly in workers in the asbestos-mining industry in South Africa and, since almost all of these had had extensive exposure to asbestos, the causal link was never in serious doubt.

Rapid recognition of the risk to people working in the asbestos industries occurred but it took longer for it to be recognized that there would be a risk to people exposed to asbestos either because they lived near to asbestos mines or because they lived in houses in which asbestos was used in the construction. Mesotheliomas were recorded in the wives and children of asbestos workers, presumably because asbestos came into the home on clothes and in the hair of the people who were exposed at work. Industrial measures to ensure showering and changing of clothes before leaving work were brought in in the 1970s.

Strict control of asbestos exposure at work and permitted asbestos levels in building are now in place.

Because of the long period of time between asbestos exposure and the development of mesothelioma, we can anticipate continuing problems. Mesothelioma is increasing in incidence in Western Europe and North America, particularly in younger patients. The prediction is that there will be a further rise through the remaining years of this century and the early part of the next century before the disease subsides in frequency as the proportion of the population who were exposed to asbestos in the early part of the century decreases.

The cause of this cancer has been identified, the means of preventing it have been put in place mainly through industrial legislation and the problem is solved. Unfortunately, because of the nature of the link between cancer and its causes many thousands of people across the world will still die of mesothelioma before the story finally closes about a quarter of the way into the next century.

Asbestos and Lung Cancer

Asbestos also increases the risk of ordinary lung cancer, although its potency in this respect is much smaller than its effect on mesothelioma. It interacts particularly with smoking in causing lung cancer. Although the effect of asbestos on the lung is much smaller than that of tobacco, it is still not trivial because of the great frequency of lung cancer. There does not seem to be the increasing incidence of lung cancer in non-smokers that we would anticipate if asbestos were a potent cause. It is probably only among smokers that the problem is significant.

Prevention of Exposure in the Workplace to Chemicals Causing Cancer

Our list above mentions a few specific chemicals which have been linked to particular cancers. A comprehensive list of chemicals which cause cancer in occupation is kept by the International Agency for Research on Cancer (IARC). The classification of chemicals which produce cancer is not, however, straightforward. The IARC categorizes chemicals according to the certainty of our knowledge: those where the link is definite (Group 1), those which probably cause cancer in humans (Group 2A), and those which possibly cause cancer in humans (Group 2B). It also keeps records of those chemicals which cannot be classified at the moment because information is insufficient.

In Table 4 we have listed the number of agents put into each category in the IARC's survey published in 1987. There are twelve industries in which chemicals are believed to cause cancer but where the precise chemical has not been identified (11 'definite' and 1 'possible'). The distribution otherwise is dominated by industrial chemicals known to be used in industrial production, either as a raw material or in some chemical synthetic process (17 'definite' and 19 'probable'). There are just 8 'probable' and 41 'possible' among chemicals which are used only for research purposes in the laboratory.

Table 4
Environmental Agents Causing Cancer

Type of agent	Causes cancer in humans	Probably causes cancer in humans	Possibly causes cancer in humans	Not known	Known to be safe	TOTAL
Industry	11	—	1	4	—	16
Industrial chemical	17	19	65	170	—	272
Pesticide	—	—	13	37	—	50
Laboratory chemical	—	8	41	67	—	116
Drug	18	10	30	71	1	129
Food ingredient	1	—	9	31	—	41
Habit	3	—	—	1	—	4
TOTAL	50	37	159	381	1	628

Table 5
Occupational Exposures Known to be a Cause of Lung and Bladder Cancer in Humans

Bladder	Lung
Aluminium production	Aluminium production
4-aminobiphenyl	Arsenic
Benzidine	Asbestos
Coal gasification	Bis(chloromethyl)ether and chloromethyl methyl ether
Coal-tar pitches	Chromium compounds (hexavelent)
Manufacture of auramine	Coal gasification
Manufacture of magenta	Coal-tar pitches
Mineral oils	Coal-tars
2-naphthylamine	Coke production
Rubber industry	Haematite mining
	Iron and steel founding
	Mustard gas (sulphur mustard)
	Nickel and nickel compounds
	Soots
	Talc containing asbestiform fibres

All this illustrates the wide variety of chemicals that are already implicated, and the fact that there are very many more which remain to be explored and characterized carefully. Work on exploring the links will continue and should be the subject of stringent controls. Detailed labelling and careful prescription of the way in which chemicals are handled in order for them to be safe is a central theme in occupational medicine and in the legislative regulation of cancer cause and chemicals. Although control of these chemicals is both expensive and time-consuming, it is essential if we are to continue to maintain our respectable record in restricting exposure in the workplace in the next century.

Where would we expect to see improvements in the overall pattern of cancer as a result of careful restriction of exposure in the workplace? The answer is probably mainly in cancers of the lung and cancer of the bladder. For these cancers, the list of possible associations with occupational exposure is probably the longest and we have illustrated the point in Table 5.

The encouraging reduction of cancers in young people in the lung and bladder which we shall discuss in detail in a later chapter is at least in part attributable to better control of cancer-causing chemicals in the workplace. The fact that this reduction is not being seen in Eastern Europe may be ominous for those countries.

Social Change and Cancer in the Workplace

We are in an era of rapid change in the workplace. In the more industrialized parts of the world, the introduction of new technology is reducing the direct involvement of workers in manufacturing and the service sectors are expanding rapidly. There is therefore a trend towards white-collar working and this trend is likely to continue or accelerate as automated processes play a greater and greater part in industry. Dr Elspeth Linge from the Danish Institute of Cancer Epidemiology in Copenhagen has recently asked whether these likely future trends will have an effect upon the incidence of cancer.

In her analysis she looks at forty-one individual kinds of cancer and compares the incidence between male skilled workers, farmers and academics living in Denmark. This sort of exercise is not very precise because there will be many other differences between these groups, besides their work environment, which might account for different rates of incidence of cancer. However, this sort of study can give us useful clues. The groups might be taken to represent the white-collared sedentary office worker (academics), the worker in industry who might be exposed to occupational hazards (skilled industrial workers) and farmers, who will typically be exposed to an outdoor environment. Many cancers showed no great difference between the different groupings in this overview. However, some cancers were more than twice as common in the skilled workers (bladder, small intestine, oesophagus, lung, liver, head and neck, breast, mesothelioma) and many of these are familiar as examples of the cancers that are related to occupational exposure. Among farmers, cancer of the lip emerged as being twice as common and this incidence is related to outdoor exposure. Among the academics, cancers of the kidney and melanoma were more than twice as common as in the other groups. Melanoma is, as discussed in Chapter 6, typically found in office workers who rush off and get sunburned for short periods on holiday and during recreation. Is there a message in this sort of analysis? It has to be interpreted cautiously because smoking will also be typical of skilled factory workers and may explain much of the excess of cancer of the head and neck, and lung cancer. Broadly, however, the study shows that skilled workers are at risk of the kinds of cancers that are associated with occupational exposures. As safety standards increase in the workplace over time, and automation reduces or replaces some of these skilled jobs, these cancers might be expected to decrease. Outdoor workers like farmers will remain at risk of the cancers associated with extensive sun exposure, for instance. The academics may represent a group whose style of working will be more common in the next century. The high incidence of melanoma in this group fits in very well with our previous suggestions and highlights the need for preventative measures in this area.

Sedentary Jobs and Exercise

The risk of cancer of the colon has been found to be greater among men in sedentary occupations than in physically active men. This finding has emerged from three case-control studies.

We do not know why this might be, but it is possible that physical activity stimulates the colon and shortens the contact between the contents of the stool and the lining of the bowel. Even when we take account of different dietary factors, the link between being sedentary and an increased risk of colon cancer still emerges. In the future, when sedentary occupations are likely to be more common, we should perhaps compensate by increasing the amount of exercise that we take.

Preventing Occupational Cancer

The general message of this chapter – and others – is that we have defined a large number of the agents to which people are exposed at work which can cause cancer. These include asbestos, chemicals used in industry and radioactivity. Cancers of the lung and bladder and leukaemia are the most obvious occupational cancers but many others may be implied. Our knowledge is incomplete but is none the less quite extensive. Preventative measures have been put in place for most of the known risks and appear to be very effective at reducing the exposure to the known cancer-causing agents. The effects of these measures may already be apparent in the falling incidence of lung and bladder cancer in young people, and we would predict that they will follow through to reduce the long-term impact of asbestos exposure. However, we are left with the aftermath of those earlier asbestos exposures which will continue to work through for decades to come. The regulations in force in the Western world are undoubtedly responsible for improvements in outlook in Western countries. We cannot be so optimistic for countries which have not taken these measures, particularly those of Eastern Europe, and occupational cancer hazards are now a major socio-economic and medical issue for those countries.

Cancer which is caused by exposure to materials in the

workplace is a numerically small problem, for which appropriate measures have already been taken. Despite our optimism, however, we need to continue to ensure that all new risks are identified early and that effective control measures are put in place rapidly. We can be optimistic about minimizing occupational cancer risks but we cannot afford to be complacent. The price for our optimism is the need for continuous vigilance.

ENVIRONMENTAL POLLUTION

When the workplace is implicated as a cause of cancer it is because the agents that cause cancer tend to be concentrated there and because people tend to go to that place regularly for a long time. However, the substances that can cause cancer in the workplace also escape into the general environment. What risk do they pose for the general population? The answer is rather similar to that for smoking. The individual who smokes is personally at very high risk; the non-smoker who lives in the same house has a higher risk of lung cancer but the effect is very much smaller. Applied to the workplace, we can say that the person who is exposed to asbestos every day in the building industry will have a very high risk of mesothelioma whereas the people who walk by the building site will have a lower risk.

The sources of pollution with which we have to be concerned are industrial processes which give rise to emissions from factory chimneys into the atmosphere, farming with pesticides and other processes which allow chemicals to enter the water, as well as sources of radiation which we have considered already in Chapter 6. How important are these general environment pollutants in the cause of cancer?

There are two separate questions that we must consider. The first is whether there are chemicals in the air or in water that are capable of causing cancer. The second is whether they occur in sufficient quantity to make any practical difference to the risk of getting cancer in the general population.

Are There Pollutants Capable of Causing Cancer in the General Environment?

The answer to this question is a very clear yes. We have already considered the International Agency for Research on Cancer categories of different chemicals in relation to the workplace. Air pollution from industrial sources can include arsenic compounds, asbestos, chromium compounds, nickel compounds, radon gas, benzene, tobacco smoke or soot, all of which are considered to be capable of causing cancer by the agency. In addition, other minerals (beryllium, cadmium, silica) and other chemicals (benzopyrene and related materials and diesel exhaust) are all considered to be *probably* capable of causing cancer, and there is a longer list of chemicals and contaminants which are *possibly* capable of causing cancer, including petrol-engine exhaust fumes. However, they are all present in very low concentration.

There is no doubt that there are tiny quantities of materials in water that can cause cancer, including chemicals, asbestos, pesticides, some of the minerals and radioactive sources. These are all part of the general background to which we are exposed.

Is There Enough Pollution to be a Significant Cause of Cancer?

The answer to this question is much less clear. Many studies have compared the incidence of cancers in city dwellers and in country dwellers. The argument runs that the city dwellers are exposed to more pollution, particularly industrial pollution. Lots of these studies have concentrated naturally on lung cancer because of its frequency and the expectation of a link to the lungs as the first organ exposed to air pollution. The studies are rather inconclusive and certainly do not suggest a very large effect of air pollution on lung cancers. Among non-smokers there is little evidence that urban dwelling is associated with a higher risk of lung cancer. There is a falling incidence of lung cancer among non-smokers, which could be related to reductions in the United Kingdom in air pollution, but the evidence is not conclusive. It seems that, for smokers, living in a polluted area may add yet further to their risk of getting lung cancer. However, the effect is small. The impact of living in an urban area or the risk of getting lung cancer is rather similar to that of passive smoking and is completely overshadowed by the effects of cigarette smoking itself.

Studies in which attempts have been made to link cancer to residence within a short distance of particular industrial plants have, in general, been unconvincing. Sometimes a higher risk of dying from lung cancer has been found for those who live near to iron and steel works or petrol and chemical plants but when the evidence is looked at more carefully it seems apparent that this effect is attributable to the high proportion of the population actually employed in those plants as their work-place, rather than to the effect of living close to the factory.

The effects of pollutants of drinking water have also been studied but the results to date are far from conclusive. Asbestos can contaminate drinking water in asbestos-mining areas and several studies have been carried out (we are aware of seven) to look at the rates of cancer in these areas compared to those in other parts of the country. There may be a slight increase in stomach cancer and pancreatic cancer but the results for most other cancer are variable and generally reassuring.

Some organic chemicals and pesticides can be found in drinking water supplies in very low concentrations. In particular, chemicals related to chloroform (so called trihalomethanes) are known to cause cancer in animals and so careful studies of the pollution of drinking water with these chemicals have been carried out and one such study reported a series of positive results in the late 1970s. However, subsequent studies have in general been very reassuring, with only the occasional worrying result. Overall, the evidence that cancer is caused by drinking-water contaminated with chemicals is pretty thin but this does not remove the need for constant vigilance because, if the concentrations of the pollutants were to increase, we would anticipate this leading to more cancers.

Some drinking water will contain radioactive materials naturally and several studies have suggested small but significant increases in cancer in people who use drinking water with slightly increased radioactivity levels in Sweden and in the United States.

CONCLUSIONS

Pollution of the environment in the air and water is not a major cause of cancer at present. However, some of the pollutants which are present in very tiny quantities are known to be capable of causing cancer in experimental situations when they are used in much higher concentrations. For this reason, we have to be continually vigilant to ensure that the quality of our air and the quality of our water is maintained.

10

Inherited Cancer – the New Genetics

We are rapidly approaching an understanding of the genetics of cancer. In modern medical and scientific practice there are a number of aspects to the study of cancer genetics. The first is about how the genes determine the make-up and behaviour of the cells when they divide. When a cell divides into two, the daughter cells inherit virtually identical copies of all the genes of the original cell. The genes are made up from DNA, which is a coding chemical, and the genes code for protein.

Molecular genetics of cancer is the study of the DNA and how these proteins work and interact, in both normal and cancerous cells, as discussed in Chapter 2.

The second aspect of genetics which relates to cancer is whether a susceptibility to cancer can be inherited from parent to child. A child inherits half of his or her genes from each parent. If there is an abnormality in either or both of these genes then this may result in an inherited disease. Diseases which are inherited in this way include cystic fibrosis and muscular dystrophy. We have a reasonably good understanding of the structure of some of the genes which are passed on from parents to children and which determine the whole biological make-up of the son or daughter. In this chapter, we want to focus on the inherited risk of cancer between generations.

The inheritance of a cancer between parents and their children is a complicated business. The first thing to say is that it is very rare for babies to be born with cancer. Even in the rare families where there is a pattern of inheritance of the disease, it normally develops at a later age. Often this will be in childhood or adolescence but, more often, inheritance of the gene leads to the development of cancer in adult life. It is therefore not the cancer itself which is passed from parents to children but rather a genetic blueprint which puts them at risk of getting a cancer. Cancer that is clearly inherited between generations is rare. However, it has an importance which is much greater than would be suggested by its rarity. Understanding the inheritance pattern leads to the possibility of preventing the onset of the cancer in the children by identifying those at risk and watching them very carefully to allow an early diagnosis or prevention. The genes that are inherited within the cancer-prone families are obviously crucially important pieces of genetic information. They determine the risk of cancer in this rare situation and if we can find out how they work we will learn a great deal about the mechanisms that underlie the development of cancer. This is already happening.

Another important aspect of inherited cancers lies in what they teach us about common cancers. The study of the pattern of inheritance of cancers in rare cancer-prone families may answer questions of relevance to commoner cancers. The common cancers are not inherited in a simple way. The chance of getting most common cancers is only slightly increased in close relatives. However, there are reasons that we will explain later for believing that there may be more to it than this and that the understanding which is gained by a study of rare disease may actually teach us about common cancers.

We intend to discuss this complicated subject in two sections. This will make things easier, but, as we have already emphasized, one of the key points is that these two sections are closely interrelated and that, for most people, the interest lies in the link between the two.

Cancer Families – the Rare Inherited Cancers

Within 'cancer families' the lifetime risk of a child born to an affected parent of developing the cancer is very high. Sometimes it may approach a 50 per cent chance and this is in keeping with what geneticists refer to as a 'dominant' inheritance pattern. It is not surprising that such diseases are rare. It would make no sense for any species to evolve while including large numbers of individuals who were massively at risk of a disease which is fatal in early life. The genetic errors that underlie the inheritance of cancers are many and varied. They consist of an abnormal structuring of a particular gene which results in the very high risk in the child if he or she is unfortunate enough to inherit that gene from the parents. Patterns of genetic inheritance are quite well understood and a skilled geneticist can work out the risks in relation to children based on the family history. This is not however an easy or straightforward task. Someone may inherit the gene and not show the illness – a situation called incomplete 'penetrance' of the gene within the family. Secondly, members of the family may die young of other causes like accidents and it may not be known whether they would ultimately have developed the disease. Some calculations of risk have to take into account how old the person is, since not all the inherited cancers occur in childhood and it may be necessary to have information about adult life to draw conclusions about whether someone carries the gene.

What sort of diseases are these inherited cancers? The list is long – over two hundred single gene disorders have been linked to such cancer. Fortunately, they are all rare. Some are associated with obvious abnormalities that exist before the cancer develops. These may be congenital, with abnormalities of the skin or the immune system being well represented and occasionally an association with certain kinds of severe learning disabilities. In the families with rare kinds of diseases of the immune system, the cancers that develop are commonly lymphomas arising from lymph glands.

In Table 6 we have listed a few examples to show the nature

Table 6
Inherited Cancers

Retinoblastoma	Tumours of eye and some others, e.g. bone tumours
Multiple endocrine neoplasia	Tumours in many hormone-producing glands
Polyposis coli	Polyps and bowel cancer
Dysplastic naevus syndrome	Unusual moles and melanoma

of these conditions. It is already possible and advisable for people from families at risk of these conditions to be carefully screened by examinations and medical tests which will help in their early diagnosis should cancers develop. The 'inherited cancer' families do not always get the same kind of cancer. Sometimes, as in retinoblastoma, there is a very characteristic site, in this case at the back of the eye, but even in this disease there are other cancers which may occur in the family. The disease called the Li–Fraumeni cancer family syndrome (after the people who described it) is associated with cancers in many different tissues, for example brain tumours, leukaemia, breast cancer or bone tumours. It is clear, therefore, that the inherited genetic abnormalities occur in many different tissues of the body and are not limited to a single site.

Modern genetics has revealed quite precisely the genetic basis of a number of these inherited cancers. Knowledge about the molecular basis of these genes now allows us to examine the DNA of individuals within the families and to predict who is at risk.

It will be possible in future to offer DNA testing to those individuals who wish to have this information about themselves. As the implications for individuals of having such testing may be serious and very varied, they require extensive counselling and support. Experience with other diseases has shown that many people will not wish to be tested.

As we learn more about the structure of the DNA responsible for the disease and the functions it determines, we may be able to understand much more about the mechanisms underlying the diseases. This may give us new ideas about prevention and cure.

The Relevance of the New Genetics for Common Cancers

The biological understanding that comes from studying the rare inherited cancers will help us to understand how common cancers are caused and work out ways of preventing them and treating them. There is, however, a point to make in relation to common cancers which is far more important.

We have already said, and will repeat here, that the vast majority of the common cancers are not inherited in any simple way. It is important that this point is understood, because this book is intended for a broad range of interested laymen and health-care professionals and it is not our purpose to sow seeds of anxiety among the children of parents who have had cancer. Cancer affects one third of the population at some time in their lives and it is important that the vast majority of these people are reassured that their children are not much more likely to be affected than the general population.

For many common cancers, however, the presence within a family of a person who has had that cancer slightly increases the risk to other members of the family. Fortunately, the effect is *small*. It is best explained by an example. Breast cancer is the commonest cause of death from cancer in women in many countries. In the United Kingdom at present the risk of a woman developing breast cancer at some time in her life is about 1 in 14. That means that of every 14 women, 1 *on average* will get breast cancer. If someone in a woman's family has already developed breast cancer and that person is a second-degree relative (that is, everyone except mother and sisters) then the woman's risk is about 1.5 times higher than that of the general population. That means that 1.5 of these women in every 14 will get breast cancer – better put as 3 in every 28 women. If the person with breast cancer in her family is a first-degree relative (mother or sister) then the risk is probably a little higher, between about 1.7 and perhaps 2.5 times. Studies in this area are not terribly precise but they do give the reader an indication of the sort of risks that are involved. There are some circumstances where the risk is much higher, and this may be the case if both the woman's mother and sister have breast cancer or if she has two sisters with breast cancer, in which circumstances her lifetime risk of getting breast cancer increases to about 1 in 4. This means that of every 4 women who have this risk, *on average* 1 will get breast cancer. This is therefore a much more substantial risk, but such multiple occurrence in one family is, fortunately, infrequent. It may be that getting breast cancer younger in life will be associated with a bigger family risk but this is not entirely clear. Similar sorts of figures exist for ovarian cancer. First-degree relatives of patients with lung cancer have a risk of developing lung cancer themselves which is a little over twice that of the general population, although of course this will be masked by the risk associated with smoking.

For colorectal (bowel) cancer, the other common cancer in the Western world, the situation is more complicated. There are a number of inherited family patterns that are associated with colorectal cancer. These are known as the 'familial polyposis syndromes', where members inherit large numbers of polyps in the bowel, some of which can become malignant. There are, however, certain other families who appear to have a very high frequency of colon cancers even when there are few polyps in the bowel. They develop multiple colon cancers at a relatively early age and may even get other cancers as well. There is therefore compelling evidence that inheritance can be a factor in bowel cancer in these rare situations. With most bowel cancer patients, however, the risk for other family members of getting the disease is not great. It is probably about twice that of the general population. Indeed, we cannot be entirely sure whether this risk is due to genetic inheritance or whether it could be due to similar patterns of diet.

It is clear therefore that, for many common cancers, there is a *small* but real increase of risk for families. This is not enough to cause alarm and despondency among the relatives of people who get cancer. They need only pay attention to the simple preventive rules that we have mapped out elsewhere in this book, which are relevant for the whole population. These figures are, however, very important to those studying the genetics of cancer.

To begin with, we should repeat here some points made above and in Chapter 2. Genes occur in pairs and we inherit one of each pair from each of our parents. If one gene in a pair is dominant, it is more likely that the biological characteristic controlled by that gene will express itself in some way and that the person carrying that gene will be affected by its presence. Let us take an imaginary gene which behaves in this dominant way and let us assume that the biological characteristic that it controls is one which will increase by 100 times the risk of cancer of a certain kind in any person who inherits that gene from a parent. If the risk for this kind of cancer in the general population were 1 in 1,000, the risk for the person carrying the imaginary gene would therefore be 1 in 10. This gene would obviously be an extremely important cancer gene and identifying it and knowing how it worked would be very valuable. The effects of such a gene can be estimated by geneticists. Their estimates are that the risk of cancer in a brother or sister of a patient who had that cancer might be two or three times the general risk, not very different from the risk for some of the common cancers. However, and perhaps most importantly, a high proportion of that type of cancer might occur in members of the population who were carriers of the gene. While there would still be a few cases of that cancer occurring in people who were not gene carriers, because the risk in the general population would remain at 1 in 1,000, the majority of people who developed that cancer would be gene carriers.

Such genes may exist. There is no hard evidence yet that they underlie any of the common cancers but the figure for the relative risk in brothers and sisters of getting a cancer is compatible with their existence.

If such genes really exist then the implications are important.

- *If we could identify the genes, we could identify the population at risk very accurately*. This means that we would know who to talk to about careful screening and preventative measures.

- *The risk within that population, who are carefully defined by knowledge of the genetic defect, is quite high*. We have defined it in our hypothetical case as being 1 in 10. This is enough of a risk to concentrate the minds of most people on the need for screening and prevention.

- *The rest of the population could be reassured and perhaps more relaxed about screening and preventative measures*. This would not only save anxiety but also save huge sums of money, because the screening procedures and the preventative education could be targeted on the high-risk population.

The search for such genes is truly a holy grail at present for scientists in cancer research. If they could be identified, then the whole process of cancer screening, prevention and management, and the risk to the whole population, could be redefined.

The practice of cancer medicine would change dramatically and the shift in emphasis for screening and prevention to high-risk groups, based on a knowledge of their genetic make-up, would be profound and effective.

It is in this area that the link between the new biology, the new genetics and screening and prevention for cancer must be made. If we can make it, then we really will be winning the war against cancer.

I I

The Mind, Society and Cancer

People are more than the sum of their chemical molecules and cells. They are social beings. As we have seen, the pattern of cancer varies from one society to another; and these different patterns reflect not only the different pool of genes in each society but also the environmental differences which may play a part in causing cancer. In this context, 'environmental differences' embrace the social, economic and political circumstances in which individuals find themselves. Such circumstances will determine many facets of their lives, including many of the physical features of their environment. Advanced industrial processes potentially expose people to more carcinogens (cancer-causing chemicals) but if the individuals who may in some way be affected by those processes happen to live in a country with a free press, pressure groups, 'watchdog' organizations and a government responsible to an electorate, there is a better chance of the necessary environmental safeguards being put in place. To take another example, prevailing social attitudes to smoking or being suntanned will have a direct influence on the extent to which individuals indulge in these risky habits. Variations in diet between countries, or between different groups within the same country, remain under investigation as a possible environmental explanation for different levels of cancer incidence. Such variations are the product of a complex web of social, economic and physical factors.

CANCER AND SOCIETY

In Chapter 3 we touched upon the sociology of cancer and, in particular, on the evidence from the United States of a higher cancer incidence in people with a low income. This was not a new observation. It had been observed in England in the 1920s that the rates of death from cancer were higher in lower socio-economic groups (less advantaged people) for many kinds of cancer. This was particularly true for stomach cancer which was very important at the time. The biggest differences in the United Kingdom at present are still seen in relation to stomach cancer, but we can also add lung cancer and cancer of the neck of the womb to those cancers which have a higher mortality in those who are less well off.

The situation is not always worse for people from a less advantaged background, however. Some cancers, such as Hodgkin's disease and testicular cancer, and, less strongly, breast cancer and ovarian cancer, are more likely to occur in wealthier people.

In 1982, Logan published a study from the International Agency for Research on Cancer called *Cancer Mortality by Occupation and Social Class*. This categorized most cancers according to the impact of socio-economic factors. We have listed some of the findings in Table 7.

Social class is therefore a powerful factor in many cancers. Why?

One argument put forward for the link was that people who are ill often experience downward movement in their social status and income. This explanation does not stand up to close examination. The length of the illness is typically too short to cause many people to change their socio-economic status.

Most of the difference is probably due to differing environmental exposures. The most powerful is probably smoking. Manual workers smoke more than professional people; typically

Table 7
Cancer and Social Class

More Deaths in Less-advantaged People	Size of the Effect
Oesophagus (gullet)	Moderate
Stomach	Large
Liver	Small
Lung	Large
Neck of the womb (cervix)	Large

More Deaths in Economically Advantaged People	
Malignant melanoma	Moderate
Breast	Small
Ovary	Small
Testis	Large
Brain	Small
Hodgkin's disease	Small

more than twice as many as in a similar age group of social classes 1 and 2. Almost all of the variation found between social classes for lung cancer, gullet cancer and head and neck cancer (which tends to occur in the same populations as lung cancer) is due to differences in smoking.

The effect of occupation will also be relevant and many of the occupational risks described in Chapter 9 are linked to particular levels of income. Manual workers are exposed to chemical toxins in the chemical and metal industries, and to asbestos in the building industry. The weak link between breast cancer and a higher socio-economic status may well be explained in part by the different timing in having children. Professional women tend to have their babies later. However, this effect is quite small and it probably does not explain fully the differences in breast cancer between different social classes.

Although we can explain only some of the differences in cancer mortality between different social classes, they are important when considering cancer prevention. The best targets for prevention are the reduction of smoking and improvements in levels of screening for cancer of the neck of the womb (cervix). The high-risk groups are those that are less well off. They still tend to be more likely to smoke and more likely to fail to attend for regular screening. Unless the preventative measures can be directed towards the high-risk parts of our society then they are doomed to be ineffective.

THE MIND AND CANCER RISK

Because the causes of cancer are not yet fully understood, it may be tempting to leap to the conclusion that cancer is psychological in origin, and we turn now to the question of the relationship between the person as a thinking and feeling being and the risk and outcome of cancer. The idea that particular personality types are more at risk of cancer is often expressed and sometimes accepted. It is a difficult theory to study scientifically. However, there have been a substantial number of attempts to approach the question in a scientific way.

Any attempt to link personality to cancer risk is made very difficult by our limited ability to accurately label or measure features of people's personalities. Psychologists have for many years sought to devise and test questionnaires that will allow individuals to be given a personality label. One of the most famous of these is Eysenck's Personality Inventory and another, from the United States, is the Minnesota Multiphasic Personality Inventory. These questionnaires seek answers to questions about attitudes and behaviour which can be analysed to produce an assessment of personality type. The questionnaires have been given to cancer patients and the results compared to those of people who do not have cancer. It is difficult to know what weight to give to the results of this kind of research because of the powerful effects on the individual of knowing that he or she has been diagnosed as having cancer. However, several studies have shown that cancer patients, when tested in this way, demonstrate a lower ability to express anger than people without cancer.

A more convincing approach has involved giving the personality questionnaires to a large number of people and then observing them over a long period of time to see which ones get cancer. Here, unfortunately, the results of the studies are far from conclusive. Some investigators have reported that people who are prone to depression are more likely to get cancer. Others have reported the reverse. We simply cannot draw convincing conclusions from the available scientific literature and the real answer to the question about the link between personality and cancer is that it remains unproven. In view of the many studies that have been done this suggests that the effect, if it is present at all, is not very large.

The other approach to a link between the mind and cancer has concentrated not so much on underlying personality type as on the things that happen to people as 'stressful life events'. Death of a loved one, disasters at work, moving house or divorce might all be regarded as adverse life events, although the element of stress they involve will vary from one individual to another. Researchers have also tried to see if the number of adverse life events is associated with a risk of getting cancer. The number of investigations that have been undertaken is substantial, and extends from the late 1960s into the 1980s. Breast cancer was a particular focus for some investigators and it is possible here to say that there is no evidence from the half dozen or so studies that have been reported that stressful life events are related to the risk of breast cancer. In other areas, including lung cancer and stomach cancer, the results are not so clear and there may be a link in these cases. Again, the real conclusion is that the link as far as most cancers is concerned is unproven. If it exists at all, it is probably not very large. This is important because a frequent question in the consultation between the cancer patient and his or her specialist is 'What did I do to bring this on myself?' Alternatively the patient may ask, 'Is this all because my husband/wife left me in the lurch?' Broadly, most cancer specialists can honestly answer 'No' to this question. Cancer does not in the main occur as a result of stressful life events. These events undoubtedly reduce the quality of life of people and are therefore important facets of their care. They are not, however, a dominant cause of cancer in our society.

THE MIND AND CANCER RECURRENCE

The relationship between personality or attitude of mind and the risk of cancer recurring after treatment is a rather different question. In this situation, the patient is already known to have had cancer which has been successfully treated. A common example would be that of a primary cancer of a breast or gastro-intestinal tract which has been removed by a surgical operation. Does the person's psychological make-up determine what happens next? The influence of attitude has been studied carefully and does seem to be important. Studies in this area were led in the United Kingdom by Stephen Greer and colleagues at King's College Hospital in London and subsequently at the Royal Marsden Hospital. They found that a woman's attitude following the removal of a breast cancer was an important determinant of the risk of recurrence. For instance, people who were characterized as having 'fighting spirit' or 'denial' did better than those who were categorized as being 'helpless and hopeless' or passive accepters of the disease. Similar links have been shown by others, although they are still difficult to study and the size of the effect is unclear. The way in which attitude might affect longer-term cancer outcome is also unknown and is the subject of subsequent studies still in progress.

Stressful Events and Recurrence

The relationship between stressful life events and relapse after a cancer operation is also the subject of active research which remains somewhat inconclusive. In a recent study conducted in Southampton over two hundred women were followed up for three and a half years after surgery for breast cancer and carefully assessed for the occurrence of stressful life events. Although over half the women reported serious emotional setbacks during this period, no major difference in recurrence was found between this group and others who had been spared such stressful events. In a previous study at Guy's Hospital, however, there did seem to be a relationship between severe interpersonal stresses and recurrence of cancer. The results were therefore conflicting. People can be reassured that relapses are not usually caused just by stress. However, stress may be a factor in some cases. Good advice probably remains that after cancer treatment people should aim to return to normal living as far as possible. It is a responsibility of the caring profession to ensure that they have access to support and counselling about stressful life events to improve their emotional quality of life and, just possibly, to reduce their risk of relapse.

We still believe that there are important interactions between mind and cancer. Although a particular personality or stressful life events do not cause cancer in a simple, direct way, the influence of mind over health remains powerful. Not only may the attitude of a patient influence the risk of relapse after breast cancer but, in general, the attitude of the patient after a diagnosis of cancer will profoundly influence his or her quality of life. The positive patient with 'fighting spirit' may well achieve more and feel better even if that cast of mind does not in every case result in a cure of the cancer.

12

Cancer and Infections – the Anti-cancer Vaccination?

Infections in man are caused by a wide range of different micro-organisms. These may be quite complicated bugs like the parasite that causes malaria or the simpler bacteria which cause many common kinds of infection like pneumonia or urine infections. The microbes that are of greatest interest to cancer research workers are called viruses. Most people are familiar with the idea of viruses which are very small and simple infectious agents causing colds or influenza or, more seriously, encephalitis or smallpox. The interest in research into viruses as a cause of cancer in man is now intensive.

The interest began with the early work that showed that viruses could cause cancers in animals. The early leader in this field was a scientist called Peyton Rous. He showed that if you took a particular kind of cancer, called a sarcoma, in a chicken and mashed it up and produced an extract from it that contained no living cells at all, and then passed it through a filter that removed known microbes like bacteria, the fluid would still cause a cancer in another chicken. The cancer caused in the other chicken was also a sarcoma. At the time it was not possible to work out the agent in the fluid that caused the cancer but similar sorts of experiments were performed on rabbits and mice. The cancers induced by this method were of many different types, including leukaemias.

From the 1950s to the 1970s there was a great interest in looking for a virus that caused cancer in humans. In general, this search was unsuccessful. As we will describe later in this chapter, viruses as a cause of human cancer are probably relatively unimportant. However, the study of viruses that might cause cancer was one of the fields of inquiry which led to the major advances of modern molecular biology.

Our understanding of how genes work and are controlled was derived from studies of viruses during the 1960s and 1970s. Finally, the discovery and study of viruses which caused cancer in animals led to the demonstration of the existence of oncogenes, genes which are present in man and which are associated with cancers. This came about because the genes that were discovered in viruses which caused cancers in animals were found to be very similar to genes that occurred normally in humans. Study of these genes, called proto-oncogenes, has given us a deeper understanding of how cancers develop. Virus biology therefore led to an important discovery in human cancer research.

What evidence is there that suggests that viruses can cause cancer in people at all?

Although the field is a complicated and fast-moving one, there are really only four areas in which viruses appear to be implicated fairly directly in the causation of human cancers:

hepatitis B virus	liver cancer
Epstein–Barr virus	lymphoma and nasopharyngeal cancer
papilloma viruses	cancer of the cervix (neck of womb)
retro-viruses	rare types of leukaemia
	AIDS (Chapter 8)

Hepatitis B

The hepatitis B virus was beginning to be understood in the early 1960s and, as its name suggests, it is a cause of hepatitis with jaundice and fever and ill health in many people all over the world. The virus can be transferred by injections, blood transfusions or sexual contact. In some parts of the world hepatitis B infection is very common and as many as 10 per cent of the population develop a state of chronic carriage of the virus in their bloodstream. Long-term infection with hepatitis B can lead to chronic hepatitis and eventually to cirrhosis. It is also clear that hepatitis B infection is strongly associated with the risk of liver cancer. In the Far East, hepatitis B is probably the main cause of liver cancer, and there are as many as 9 million cases of liver cancer in China every year.

Perhaps the clearest study linking hepatitis B virus with liver cancer was performed in Taiwan in the late 1970s and reported in 1981. In this study, patients with hepatitis B infection were followed up for many years, and it was found that the chance of getting liver cancer was 217 times higher in the virus-infected group than in people who were not infected with the virus. Not only that, but more than half the deaths that occurred in patients who had hepatitis B infection were caused by liver disease such as cirrhosis or liver cancer. In the population who were not infected very few developed cirrhosis or liver cancer.

Epstein–Barr Virus

Epstein–Barr virus was discovered during studies of a rare kind of lymphoma which occurs in east Africa and which was described by the British surgeon Denis Burkitt in 1958. This lymphoma occurred in a restricted area of tropical Africa, and Burkitt suggested that this might be because of a virus infection. In 1964, virus particles were discovered in cells that had been grown from patients with Burkitt's lymphoma and this virus was found to be of the family known as herpes viruses (although it is quite different from the common herpes viruses that cause cold sores). The virus is named after the two British researchers who first identified it.

Infection with Epstein–Barr virus, particularly in the Western world, results in an unpleasant but self-limiting condition called glandular fever or infectious mononucleosis. For reasons that are still not entirely understood, the infection persists in African patients, perhaps as a result of other assaults upon these patients by infections like malaria, and can lead eventually to the development of the lymphoma. We know that the tumour cells of Burkitt's lymphoma have particular rearrangements of their DNA which bring oncogenes into a form of activity that is capable of turning the cell into a lymphoma cell.

Apart from its well-established role as one of the elements causing Burkitt's lymphoma, Epstein–Barr virus has also been linked to cancer occurring at the back of the nose and throat, nasopharyngeal carcinoma, which is quite common in some parts of China and Africa. Exactly how Epstein–Barr virus causes nasopharyngeal cancer in these areas is not clear, but the association seems to be quite strong.

Finally, patients who have long-standing deficiency of their immune system, including those with AIDS, can develop lymphomas. It appears that, at least in some cases, the Epstein–Barr virus is the cause, probably again because the patients cannot get rid of the virus from their bodies and its persistence leads to the lymphoma.

Papilloma Viruses

Warts on the hands or feet (verrucae) are in fact a simple kind of tumour. They are not malignant and therefore must not be confused with cancers. They result from the proliferation of cells as a result of an infection with viruses called papilloma viruses.

There is a fair amount of evidence that suggests a role for papilloma viruses in cancer of the neck of the womb (cervix) in women. This is discussed in Chapter 8; the evidence is mostly the presence of the virus and its active genes within the cells of the cancer of the cervix. Papilloma virus infections probably cause the changes in cells of the cervix which we call dysplasia and which are detected by cervical screening. Approximately 70 per cent of all cancers of the cervix appear to contain DNA derived from certain kinds of papilloma viruses. Infection with papilloma viruses alone is not sufficient to cause cancer. Most individuals who are infected do not get cancers and other factors need to operate. Smoking appears to be associated with cancer of the cervix and it may be that the chemicals that get into the bloodstream from smoking are sufficient to act together with the virus to produce this cancer.

Retro-viruses

The viruses that cause a rare kind of leukaemia are known as retro-viruses. This type of virus is common among those viruses that cause cancers in animals. Very few retro-viruses appear to cause cancers in man, but during the 1980s it became clear that a rare kind of leukaemia, found mainly in Japan but also occasionally in the Caribbean and with rare cases in Europe and North America, is due to infection of blood lymphocytes by a leukaemia-causing retro-virus.

A great deal of the molecular biology of these viruses is understood and the way in which they can produce these rare leukaemias is also understood. It does not seem that viruses of this kind cause, in any direct way, the commoner kinds of leukaemia found in Europe and North America.

PREVENTION OF INFECTIONS WHICH CAUSE CANCER

Avoiding infectious agents can be a very effective way of avoiding the cancer that they may cause. Unfortunately, such avoidance is not easy for hepatitis B virus or Epstein–Barr virus because they are very common in the environments where they cause problems. Similarly in those parts of the world where the retro-virus-induced leukaemias occur, the disease is transferred within communities. However, the transmission of papilloma viruses, which have been linked to cancer of the cervix, can be reduced if people cut down the number of their sexual contacts.

Greater interest has focused on the development of vaccines which might serve to immunize people against these viruses and therefore avoid the long-term infection which can lead to cancers. Vaccines are not yet at all practical for retro-viruses or papilloma viruses and are still in the very early stages of development for Epstein–Barr virus. However, effective vaccines for hepatitis B do now exist and are routinely used to avoid hepatitis in people such as doctors and nurses who work with potentially infectious sources. This approach, involving widescale vaccination against hepatitis B, is probably one way of reducing the incidence of liver cancer in China and most parts of Africa where it is common. Perhaps the biggest problem is really one of public health – the difficulty of establishing good vaccination programmes and the costs of establishing them. Nevertheless, in these particular limited cases, the possibility of vaccination as a means of avoiding cancer is a very real one.

13

Screening for Cancer

We have talked so far about the nature of cancer, its cause and prevention. In this chapter we are going to examine another approach, which has become known as cancer screening. The principle here is quite different. The aim is to make the diagnosis of a cancer very early in its life or even when it is at a stage leading up to the cancer, known as pre-malignancy. Treatment given at this time might be expected to be more likely to produce a cure than treatment given later in the course of the illness, when the disease is larger or has spread to distant parts of the body.

The attraction of screening for cancer has been apparent for many decades and a wide range of approaches has been taken to many different cancer sites. In the United Kingdom screening has now achieved established status as the major approach to reducing deaths from breast cancer and cancer of the neck of the womb (cervix) in women. Before considering the basis of this approach and its value, it is worth pausing to consider the underlying scientific ideas of screening.

Screening and Cancer Biology

The diagram overleaf shows a simplified model of how cancers grow and spread. If we just think of the local cancer growing at its primary site we can imagine it as starting off as a very small bunch of cells, which gradually increase in number until it reaches a size that is large enough to be detected either by the patient or by the doctor on examination. This is the stage of clinical diagnosis. At this point, if it is not effectively

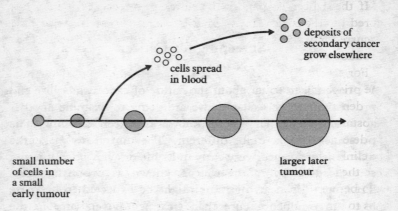

cells spread
in blood

deposits of
secondary cancer
grow elsewhere

small number
of cells in
a small
early tumour

larger later
tumour

Figure 17 The natural history of a cancer.

removed, it will continue to grow, causing steadily more and more problems for the patient until, ultimately, if it gets big enough or invades far enough, it can prove fatal. Meanwhile, somewhere along the course of the growth of that cancer, bits will break off and spread to distant parts of the body. We have already discussed this process in Chapter 2 but it is worth repeating some of the points. Once that process of breaking off and spreading to distant parts of the body has occurred the cancer will not be cured by a local operation or by radiotherapy to the primary site. It will only be cured if we have effective drugs that go everywhere in the body and pick up all of the deposits that have spread through the bloodstream. Effective drugs are only available for a minority of cancers, so the process of spread, or metastasis, is associated with a very poor outcome, usually fatal.

If the cancer is diagnosed before spread occurs it may be cured by a local treatment. If it is diagnosed after spread has occurred no amount of local treatment can be expected to produce a cure.

For screening to work we have to have a means of detecting the primary cancer before it has spread, and we have to be able to demonstrate that it can be detected at this stage in a substantial number of people. The screening test has to be able to detect the cancer earlier in its growth pattern than the point of clinical diagnosis. If it cannot do that, we might as well wait for the clinical diagnosis to be made. Most importantly, the gap between the screening diagnosis and the clinical diagnosis has to include the point where the tumour starts to spread. If it does not, there will be no benefits from screening. If spread occurs before the screening test can detect the cancer, then screening is too late and no extra cures will be achieved. If spread occurs after the clinical diagnostic point then there is no point in making the early diagnosis by screening because you will get just as many cures at the point of clinical diagnosis. This is illustrated in Figure 18.

It is worth pointing out that screening can have other benefits as well as increasing the cure rate. Early diagnosis usually means that the treatment can be given locally without such big operations or such extensive radiotherapy. This has many benefits for the patient because these treatments are often unpleasant and may produce local damage or mutilation. A spin-off from screening is therefore a reduction in the severity of the treatment that is required. However, the principal goal of screening is to increase the cure rate.

The explanations and the diagrams should make the point that we cannot just assume that screening works. We need to have some means of testing it. We can do this by comparing its

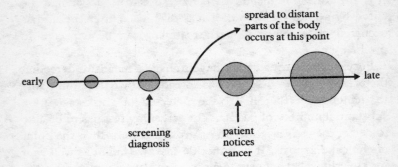

Figure 18 (a) Screening works.

In this situation screening works. The screening test makes the diagnosis before the tumour has spread and a simple operation leads to a cure.

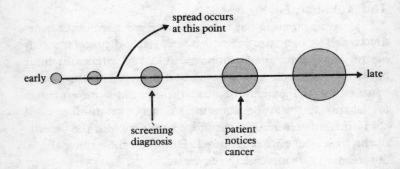

Figure 18 (b) Screening fails.

Even when screening makes the diagnosis, spread has already occurred – screening fails and the patient's chances are poor.

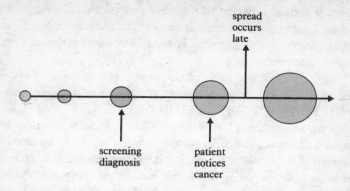

Figure 18 (c) Screening cannot help.

Spread would have occurred late in this case, after the patient has consulted the doctor. Screening would not have helped here and the patient should do well.

effectiveness in one group of people against some sort of control population. We also need to have an understanding of the biology of the disease that guarantees that the screening test will make the diagnosis in many patients before there is any chance of spread. The two most important screening exercises in the United Kingdom are based on these two principles.

For breast cancer there have been, over the last two or three decades, a number of studies which have compared the effects for one group which was offered screening with the outcome for a control group of women who were not screened, This has produced evidence that screening works. This means that there is indeed a period of time before the clinical diagnosis of breast cancer during which spread of the cancer occurs. It also means that the screening test is capable of making the diagnosis before that spread occurs.

For cancer of the neck of the womb (cancer of the cervix) the principle is a little different. In this case, the diagnosis is made by taking a sample of cells from the neck of the womb and smearing them on a glass slide which is stained and examined under the microscope. These cells can be used to make the diagnosis of an early cancer, but more often, changes in their appearance will tell the person carrying out the test that they are not yet cancer but are likely to turn into cancer cells. This is an example of a pre-malignant lesion and we know that quite a lot of these pre-malignant lesions will progress to invasive cancer at some time in the future. Screening allows us to make the diagnosis before that occurs and therefore to reduce the occurrence of that cancer and the number of people who die of it.

These two examples seem quite straightforward when described in this way. In fact the history of the subject is far from straightforward. For many years controversy raged between doctors and scientists who believed that spread of breast cancer occurred so early in its course that screening would never work and others who believed that the spread did not occur so early. As is so often the case, neither side was entirely right. There is, it seems, only a relatively narrow 'window' into which screening has to fit in order to be effective.

Even with cancer of the cervix a great deal of controversy raged for a long time. There was great debate as to whether the abnormalities that we now call pre-malignant in the neck of the womb actually did lead on to cancer. In many countries doctors and scientists doubted this possibility and it took decades of careful work for everyone to be convinced.

The Pitfalls of Screening

It might be thought reasonable at first to believe that it would only be necessary to look at the outcome of cancer in patients whose diagnosis was made at screening to find out whether it was effective. If such patients did well, that would support the case for screening everybody. In fact this is not true. There are a whole series of factors that can be misleading. It is worth illustrating some of these to point out how difficult it is to arrive at any certainty in this area. The first is so-called lead-time bias. If you consider Figure 18a it is clear that the screening diagnosis is made earlier than the clinical diagnosis. If the gap between the two is one year then you might expect every patient diagnosed by screening to live a year longer on average after the diagnosis than the patients diagnosed in the clinic. It should therefore surprise nobody if survival after the screening diagnosis is longer than survival after a clinical diagnosis, and this by itself does not prove the effectiveness of screening. Indeed, unless spread actually fits in between the two diagnostic times as in Figure 18a, all that you have achieved by screening is giving the patient the information that they have a cancer a year earlier, and that may not be a service at all. So this source of bias – known as lead-time bias – has to be borne in mind when conducting studies. There are other kinds of bias that can give a falsely favourable impression of screening. Screening is more likely to make the diagnosis in tumours which take a very long time to grow, and these are already associated with a good outcome. Screening will make the diagnosis in those patients who tend to come forward and be screened and, at the moment, these tend to be the healthier and wealthier segments of the community whose outcome, in any case, is often better than the poorer, less generally healthy members of our community. Finally, screening will bring to light a host of very early abnormalities and it is not certain that all of these will turn into cancer. If they are counted as cancers, then the success rate attributed to screening might again be falsely reassuring.

All of these sources of bias have to be kept in mind. It is not enough to show that screening makes the diagnosis earlier. That is in itself not surprising. The case for screening must rest on its capacity to make a correct diagnosis at a time that will allow curative treatment and lead to a decreased death rate from the cancer screened.

The World Health Organization has indicated its views on the place of screening programmes. They believe screening programmes are appropriate if the disease being screened for is common and serious, the test is accurate and safe, and there is evidence that the test makes the diagnosis at an appropriate time, when cures can be achieved. They point out that there has to be an acceptable treatment for it to be worth making the diagnosis.

SCREENING FOR CANCER OF THE CERVIX

Screening for cancer of the cervix is potentially highly effective. The existence of a well-characterized pre-malignant lesion which can be detected by taking cells from the neck of the womb and examining them under a microscope makes this potentially the most effective of all known screening tests. When the sample of cells from the cervix is examined, the risk of them turning into cancer can be estimated. If they are normal, no risk is present. If they are very abnormal the risk may be high. However, between these extremes there are differing degrees of abnormality. Mild degrees of abnormality may indicate an increased risk of cancer, but some of these minor abnormalities do not progress to cancer and some may do so very, very slowly. We want to emphasize that an abnormal smear test is *not* the same as a diagnosis of cancer. It may often only mean that measures need to be taken to make sure that the woman does *not get cancer*. This is true and effective prevention.

Perhaps the most compelling evidence for the effectiveness of well-organized screening programmes comes from Scandinavia. Such programmes were introduced in Iceland, Finland and Sweden, and they resulted in a gradual reduction in the incidence of cancer of the cervix. In Denmark the services were less well organized and the effect was a little less. Norway did not introduce a proper programme of screening at the same time and there was little fall in cancer of the cervix.

Similar observations were made in Canada. In the United Kingdom the results are far from satisfactory. Screening has been operated in the United Kingdom since 1964 but it is hard to detect any substantial effect. It has, however, been claimed that screening might have resulted in halting an increase in cervical cancer that would otherwise have occurred. The main difference between the successful Scandinavian programmes and the UK is that in Scandinavia every eligible woman was personally invited to be screened at regular intervals and 80 per cent or more accepted, whereas in the UK there was no organized invitation system.

In 1987, a working party of doctors and scientists in the United Kingdom examined the results of screening and decided that a series of recommendations should be implemented to ensure that the benefits of screening were available to the United Kingdom population. They recommended that all women aged between twenty and sixty-four should be personally invited to attend for screening and that there should be considerable educational input to ensure that the women at greatest risk came forward for screening. They also emphasized the importance of putting in place appropriate laboratory and administrative support for the screening programme. The Department of Health has instructed all health authorities to

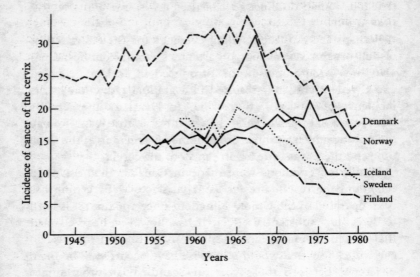

Figure 19 Trends in the annual age-adjusted incidence rates of invasive carcinoma of the cervix.

The trends in the incidence of cancer in different Scandinavian countries reflect their use of screening. In Norway the system was poor and the reduction in incidence was also poor, as shown above; only about 10 per cent of deaths were avoided between 1965 and 1982. In Iceland, Finland and Sweden the screening was much more effective. Eighty per cent of the eligible population was screened and the incidence of cancer was reduced impressively. In Denmark only 40 per cent of the eligible population was screened. As a result of the fall in incidence, deaths from cancer of the cervix were reduced by 80 per cent (Iceland), 50 per cent (Finland), 34 per cent (Sweden) and 25 per cent (Denmark) between 1965 and 1982. In these countries, well-organized screening programmes had a dramatic effect in reducing cancer deaths.

(Prepared from data provided by the Cancer Research Campaign Factsheet, 'Cervical Cancer Screening'.)

develop programmes that will call and recall the appropriate women for screening, and offered general practitioners incentive payments for screening a high proportion of their women patients. It remains a challenge to see whether in the United Kingdom we can match the level of organization that was achieved in parts of Scandinavia.

It is now recognized that the best way to organize the screening programme involves a system for routinely inviting women, using computerized family practice lists, together with high quality control when taking smears and reading them. The targeting of the population must be organized in such a way that screening reaches women from all social groups. It is not sufficient to provide screening which will only be taken up by well-educated and wealthy women who may be at a lower risk of this disease anyway. A wide age band has to be approached. Just screening people during family planning and maternity clinics is ineffective because cervical cancer is much commoner in older women.

The number of tests to be done and their frequency has to be very carefully judged. The effect of varying the frequency of screening by cervical smears can be calculated. If cervical smears are done every five years from the age of twenty to the age of sixty-five it is possible to predict that the reduction in the rate of cancer of the cervix will be some 84 per cent. If the frequency is increased to every three years the reduction is over 90 per cent and if screening is done every year the reduction is 93 per cent. On the other hand, very frequent screening means many more tests, with associated discomfort and anxiety and cost to the health service. Frequent tests may be acceptable to the very committed members of society who take up screening anyway and who tend to be at lowest risk. However, they may not be so attractive to those less-committed individuals who need to be reached by screening if it is to be effective. The middle road therefore seems sensible and cost effective. Screening every three to five years from the age of twenty to the age of sixty-five will reduce the incidence of invasive cancer of the cervix by over 80 per cent, a remarkable achievement for a relatively simple procedure.

The high priority which should be given to appropriate screening for cervical cancer is recognized by doctors, scientists and by the government. Its proper implementation will be one of the best indicators of the success of the National Health Service in the next decade.

Among the failings of the earlier efforts in the United Kingdom were a lack of communication with women and the failure to invite them to be screened. Recent more concerted efforts in most health districts include careful attention to providing information to family doctors and to women. Best practice demands that women are told when they should be screened and then when they might expect to be informed of the result and whom to contact if they do not receive information within that time limit.

SCREENING FOR BREAST CANCER

Breast cancer is one of the most important medical problems in the United Kingdom. There are almost 25,000 new cases every year and 15,000 deaths. Breast cancer accounts for 5 per cent of all deaths in women in the United Kingdom and is the commonest cause of death of women in middle age. The United Kingdom has almost the highest breast cancer mortality of any country which keeps records.

Breast cancer occurs in an organ which is easily examined. When the cancer is small it can be removed without much surgical damage to the breast. This would suggest that early diagnosis of the kind achieved by screening might result in a useful outcome in that the cancer would be easily treated and the patient might be readily cured. However, we have already discussed the reasons for caution in believing that early diagnosis would necessarily lead to cure and it has required many decades of work to establish the curative potential of screening in breast cancer.

The evidence that screening *can* lead to an increased cure rate in breast cancer and reduce the overall mortality in the population is now very strong. Three countries (the United States, Sweden and Scotland) have performed trials in which a population of women were either screened or not according to the study design. The first study was carried out in New York using methods of clinical examination and breast X-rays (mammograms) and screening women between forty and sixty-four years of age every year. The second was carried out in Sweden and used mammography alone in women over the age of forty every eighteen months to three years. Both studies showed a reduction in mortality of about 30 per cent compared to mortality in the control group. It remains difficult to be precise about the size of the benefits. In the age group 50–69 years, the deaths from breast cancer are probably reduced by between 20 and 30 per cent if screening is introduced to the population. If an individual woman of this age goes for screening her personal risk of dying from breast cancer in the next ten years may be reduced by more than this – perhaps 40 per cent. Slightly less rigorous studies have been carried out in Italy and the Netherlands using the case-control method. They all used mammography but the ages of patients studied differed somewhat. Screening was at between one- and four-yearly intervals. The studies also showed a reduction in mortality compared to that of the unscreened population. All this evidence is pretty compelling. Screening for breast cancer is feasible and can be effective.

This is not all that we need to consider. We have to ask who should be screened, how often they should be screened and by what technique. The evidence suggests that the benefits are greatest for women over the age of fifty. The benefit of screening women below fifty is uncertain and further research will be necessary before screening can be firmly recommended for women under that age. Mammography seems to be a necessary part of a successful screen. As we shall explain, breast examination alone is insufficient. It seems as though screening has to be carried out at least every three years.

The obvious screening test is for a doctor or other health-care professional to examine the breast. It is difficult by this method to pick up cancers that are smaller than about 1 cm and many lumps that are not cancer will be detected. Examination by itself is therefore potentially rather insensitive and most evidence to date suggests that this approach is insufficient. Mammography is a technique that uses very small doses of X-rays to produce a picture of the breast which is much more sensitive than physical examination and can give useful information about whether the abnormalities seen are due to a cancer or are not. The radiation dose is tiny and mammography is at present the most sensitive technique for finding a breast cancer in screening.

In 1988 Health Authorities in the United Kingdom began phasing in the National Breast Screening Programme. A nationwide service is being established to apply mammography every three years to women aged between fifty and sixty-four years. This is a huge and expensive undertaking but it can potentially reduce the death rate from breast cancer by one quarter in this age group. There remain arguments about the cost-effectiveness of the programme and the possible anxieties provoked by screening. Nevertheless it is a major health initiative and deserves support.

SCREENING FOR OTHER CANCERS

Screening programmes for breast and cervix cancers are the only established procedures at present.

Screening for cancers other than these is not yet of proven value but there is considerable potential for a possible reduction of deaths from some cancers in future. Perhaps the most promising areas are cancer of the bladder and cancer of the bowel (colorectal), cancer of the stomach in high-risk populations, melanoma by skin examinations and possibly ovarian cancer by blood tests and ultrasound when the tests improve.

Lung Cancer

Screening for lung cancer by chest X-rays and looking for cancer cells in the sputum has proved uniformly disappointing, and a number of studies have shown that there is no improvement in survival. This is therefore not to be routinely recommended: there is not sufficient reason for routine chest X-rays or for including chest X-rays in medical examinations for screening purposes.

Bowel Cancer

Screening for colorectal (bowel) cancer is more promising but has not yet been fully evaluated. Cancers in the bowel bleed slightly at a very early stage. Such blood may not be visible in the stool but can be detected by sensitive chemical reactions known as occult blood tests. Large-scale trials are in progress to find out if the use of occult blood tests will detect bowel cancers early enough to have an impact on the mortality from this disease. It is already becoming clear that using the occult blood tests results in the diagnosis of cancer being made at an earlier stage. It is not yet clear, however, that there is a survival advantage to be obtained and the results of further research must be awaited.

Bladder Cancer

Bladder cancer can be detected by examining the urine for cells shed by the cancer. It is not, however, clear that such a technique will reduce the mortality from bladder cancer. Screening for bladder cancer achieves greater importance in high-risk populations and these are found particularly in countries where the bladder infestation schistosomiasis is widespread. This is a particular problem in Egypt. In developed countries populations at particular risk would include those exposed to industrial agents which might put them at a higher risk of bladder cancer. Again, routine screening cannot be recommended at the present time.

Ovarian Cancer

Cancer in the ovary can be detected by a blood test measuring a material called CA125 and by ultrasonic scanning. Again, it is not clear that these tests will result in a reduced mortality from this disease. So far the results of screening for ovarian cancer have been disappointing, but there is a need for further studies in this area as new techniques which are more sensitive at detecting the disease become available.

Stomach Cancer

In Japan, screening for stomach cancer by X-rays has produced some evidence for a reduction in mortality but it is hard to distinguish this effect from an overall fall in incidence of stomach cancer which is occurring anyway. A big problem with stomach cancer screening is that it is very expensive. Initial X-ray examinations often need to be followed by a gastroscopy, quite a minor procedure in itself – the stomach is examined through a fibre-optic telescope – but expensive to perform on very large numbers of people. The value of screening for stomach cancer must depend on how frequent the disease is in the screened population, and it is probably only going to be practical to consider this in places such as Japan or Latin America with a very high incidence.

—

CAN SCREENING CAUSE HARM?

There must be some potential for harm in screening if it is not very carefully organized and if judgements about its use are not carefully made. Many people must be screened in order to save one life. Screening is potentially very expensive and, in a health service with finite resources, will compete with other health measures. If the screening test is not specific for the cancer, lots of people may be alarmed by the need to have further tests and these may often in fact be unnecessary and result only from the lack of specificity of the screening test. We do not know whether the anxiety raised will do psychological harm to the people screened.

All this argues for careful and cautious introduction of screening, but it does not argue against the introduction of screening. We need to look for evidence of specificity and we need to look for evidence of psychological harm. If we find such evidence, then screening programmes may need to be modified. This need for caution has to be set against the possibility of dramatically reducing the incidence of the potentially fatal cancer in the cervix and significantly reducing the mortality from breast cancer.

THE FUTURE OF SCREENING

Screening is likely to be an important part of health-promotion programmes into the next century. Cancer of the cervix and cancer of the breast are major causes of death in women and have so far yielded only slightly to other approaches to reduce their mortality. Unless effective drug treatment for established disease is discovered or effective prevention becomes possible, early diagnosis by screening is our best chance of reducing the effect of these diseases. Large-bowel cancer may be the next to yield but we shall have to await the results of studies now in progress before we can be sure. It is to be hoped that further advances in our knowledge of the causes of cancers will allow us to recognize who is most at risk and concentrate the screening methods for any cancer as they become available on those people who have most to gain.

14

How Much Cancer is Preventable?

We have now discussed all the important causes of cancer. The reader will have an idea of certain powerful factors like smoking that clearly cause cancer and are still relatively uncontrolled, and of the opportunities that seem to be emerging for minimizing risks through the study of diet as a cause. The importance of sunburn, radiation, sex, hormones, reproduction, workplace exposure, infections and the importance of inherited risk factors have been examined. Which are the most important and where do we go from here?

In 1981 Richard Doll and Richard Peto from Oxford looked at what was known or suspected about cancer cause and made some estimates of the importance of the different factors.

Figure 20 gives an idea of the contributions which seem likely to be made by the different factors we have discussed. There is still uncertainty about diet as a cause of cancer although, as we indicated in the relevant chapter, it may well be very important. In their original paper, Doll and Hill suggested diet might account for some 35 per cent of cancer overall, and in a recent paper in 1992, Sir Richard Doll still held to that estimate and felt that changes in diet patterns in the USA might be contributing to lower rates for some cancers in young people. Some questions and doubts are left in the diagram but a few things are very clear.

Smoking is the dominant cause of cancer in the Western world and far outweighs any other known factor. Some 30 per cent of cancer deaths are due to smoking and these are mainly lung cancer but include the other cancers discussed in Chapter 4. Compared with smoking, the contributions of alcohol, work-

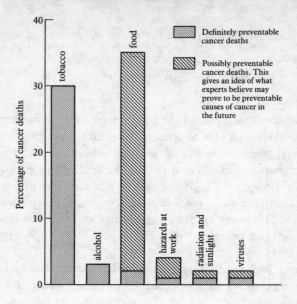

Figure 20 Percentage of cancer deaths by cause.

(Prepared from data provided by the Cancer Research Campaign, based on Doll, R., and Peto, R., *The Causes of Cancer*, Oxford University Press, 1981.)

place hazards, radiation, sunburn and virus infections are pretty small. Even if we accept the evidence that virus infection causes cancer of the cervix, which is now much stronger than when Doll and Peto wrote their paper, the figures do not change a great deal.

Another important feature of these numbers justifies comment. When they are all added up, even with the uncertainty about the importance of diet, it is clear that we know the cause of more than half of cancer deaths and that we might prevent most of these. This is really the message of this book. Causes are known and prevention is readily available for many human cancers.

Table 8
Causes of Cancers and Deaths in the United Kingdom

Cancer	Definite cause	Probable cause	Deaths in 1985 in UK
Bladder	Tobacco, chemicals	—	5,358
Brain	—	—	2,940
Breast	Hormones	—	15,381
Cervix	—	Viruses	2,170
Colon and rectum	—	Diet	19,452
Gullet	Alcohol and smoking	—	5,591
Ovary	—	Hormones	4,275
Kidney	—	Tobacco	2,667
Leukaemia	Radiation	—	4,084
Liver	Alcohol, viruses	—	1,607
Lung	Tobacco	Radon	40,223
Lymphoma	—	Viruses	3,921
Melanoma	Sunburn	—	1,192
Pancreas	—	Smoking	6,797
Prostate	—	—	8,234
Stomach	—	Diet	10,612
All cancers			162,558

In Table 8 we have listed the cancers that cause more than one thousand deaths every year in the United Kingdom, together with their known or probable causes. It is quite clear that we know a lot about the cause of most of them.

HOW MUCH OF EACH KIND OF CANCER IS PREVENTABLE?

A theoretical approach that can be taken towards estimating how much of each kind of cancer might be prevented by careful measures was taken by Tomatis and his colleagues in their excellent book *Cancer: Causes, Occurrence and Control*, produced by International Agency for Research on Cancer Scientific Publications in 1990. For each site of cancer they estimated the frequency of that cancer in the highest-risk area in the world compared to the frequency in a lower-risk area and tried to match up areas in which the populations have a rather similar racial, ethnic and therefore genetic, background. The difference was then assumed to be due to the exposure of the high-risk population to risk factors in the environment. Since environmental risk factors are frequently (but not always) correctable, the difference between the two regions provided a measure of the proportion of cancers which could be considered environmental and which *might* then be prevented.

It is worth going through each cancer site because it does give us an idea of the potential power of cancer prevention. We must emphasize that this does not mean that these preventative measures can be switched on easily because, in many cases, the precise environmental causes for any particular cancers in any particular high-risk area are not fully understood. The exception of course is lung cancer and smoking, but we have already made that point quite emphatically. The following sections give the reader an impression of the extent to which each cancer might be prevented if we knew all the causative factors in the environment and could do something about them.

Cancer of the Mouth

In certain areas of France the incidence rates for mouth cancer are eight times those in certain areas of Spain and the ethnic population is similar. This gives us an estimated preventable rate of 83 per cent. The important factors are alcohol, smoking and chewing tobacco, and these are all avoidable.

Cancer of the Stomach

The highest-risk area is Japan and the lowest-risk area is Kuwait and the difference is some twentyfold; the genetic background of the two races is of course quite different. There is a steady downward trend in gastric cancer all over the world and this almost certainly indicates a reduction in exposure to important agents in food or perhaps the introduction of some protective elements in food. We do not know exactly what these elements are, so the potential for maximizing the prevention of stomach cancer in Japan is limited, even though theoretically it approaches 90 per cent.

Bowel Cancer

There are large differences between North America, Western Europe and New Zealand, which have a high incidence of bowel cancer, and Africa, where the incidence is low, but many factors influence this. Calculations suggest that between 30 and 50 per cent of colorectal cancers might be prevented by modifications of diet to include more fibre and vegetables, and possibly by a reduction in fat or cooked meat intake.

Cancer of the Liver

Huge variations in liver cancer occur between Western countries and those of southern Africa and south-east Asia, and these are believed to be due largely to higher rates of infection with hepatitis B virus in the latter. Dietary elements, including aflatoxin from a fungus which grows on food, may also be an important contributory factor in some countries. The potential preventability of cancer of the liver derived by comparing the higher with the lowest incidence rates is over 90 per cent and most of this is likely to be achieved on a worldwide basis by effective hepatitis B vaccination. The best estimates for the effects of vaccination suggest that, with full vaccination of most newborns, the reduction in the incidence could be 65 per cent in high-risk areas.

Variations in incidence of liver cancer between Western countries are likely to be caused partly by different patterns of alcohol consumption, and the effect of reducing alcohol intake would be substantial (probably of the order of 20 to 40 per cent).

Cancer of the Pancreas

Cancer of the pancreas is three times as common in parts of Switzerland as it is in parts of Spain and the estimated potential for prevention is some 70 per cent. However, we do not know enough about the causes of pancreatic cancer to turn that into reality at this stage. The only consistent factor which emerges is an association between pancreatic cancer and tobacco smoking: estimates of the proportion of the cases that are due to smoking vary between 13 and 50 per cent. Certainly a significant proportion of cancer of the pancreas could be reduced by measures to reduce smoking although the effect is much smaller than for lung cancer.

Lung Cancer

The very large proportion of lung cancer deaths (90 per cent) that would be avoided by giving up smoking was indicated in Chapter 4. The benefits are seen some five years after giving up, although in very heavy smokers there is a further reduction in risk occurring after ten years. Realizing these benefits will be hard work. The largest study so far attempted, in which a community was intensively educated about dietary and smoking habits by public-health education and by reorganizing community health services, was carried out in Karelia in Finland and involved 180,000 people. By comparison with the rates for cancers in other parts of Finland it has been estimated that, after fourteen years, there has been a 10 per cent reduction in lung cancer. We still have a long way to go to realize the 90 per cent reduction in lung cancer which would be achieved eventually if tobacco smoking disappeared completely.

Malignant Melanoma of the Skin

If we compare white people in the United Kingdom with white people in Australia, we see that the rates of melanoma differ so greatly that about 90 per cent of Queensland's melanoma is potentially preventable. The exact achievements that are possible by reducing people's risk of sunburn are much harder to estimate and figures in the order of 40 or 50 per cent are suggested. It is unlikely that we would reduce the risk of melanoma by as much as 90 per cent, even with the most careful attention to avoiding sunburn.

Breast Cancer

The highest rate of breast cancer recorded in women of European origin is in the San Francisco Bay area of the United

States, whereas the lowest is in Poland, and the calculations suggest that almost 80 per cent of the breast cancer in California is potentially preventable. Estimates comparing Japanese living in Japan with those living in San Francisco give a figure for the proportion of preventable breast cancer of some 60 per cent. We do not know yet what are the necessary changes that would lead to this reduction in breast cancer. Changes in reproductive patterns may be a factor and diet is potentially important, although its role has not yet been clarified. Alcohol consumption may be a small factor. A realistic estimate of the possible prevention of breast cancer by hormonal and diet changes in future, on the basis of increased knowledge, might be 30 per cent.

Cancer of the Neck of the Womb (Cervix)

Most deaths from cancer of the cervix can be prevented by screening. Other forms of prevention have a smaller role and are not well defined. Changing sexual practices, vaccination against papilloma virus and reduction of cigarette smoking may all be helpful, but should not take the focus away from the major results that could be achieved by an effective screening programme.

Cancer of the Ovary

Variations in risks across Europe lead to calculations that suggest that up to 65 per cent of cancer of the ovary might be prevented. Hormonal manoeuvres like combined oral contraceptives reduce ovarian cancer risk by as much as 40 per cent, and it is in this area that the potential for prevention may lie. There are however disadvantages in the use of oral contraceptives, and their routine use as a preventive measure for ovarian cancer is not recommended.

Cancer of the Prostate

Calculations suggest that 70 or 80 per cent of cancer of the prostate is potentially preventable but we do not know yet enough about the risk factors to have a clear picture of how this can be done.

Cancer of the Bladder

Here, the potential for prevention is similarly great, and may exceed 80 per cent. We know that smoking is an important factor and estimates vary around about the 50 per cent mark for the proportion of bladder cancer that would be prevented by reducing smoking. In countries with a high rate of bladder infestation with schistosomiasis, like Iraq, Egypt and Malawi, the potential for prevention of bladder cancer by controlling the infestation is often over 50 per cent. Infection with the schistosome also gives rise to a different disease, called bilharzia, which is caught by drinking or bathing in water which contains snails carrying this parasite. In parts of Egypt the prevalence of infection with schistosomiasis has been reduced from almost 50 per cent of the population to under 10 per cent, but it will be a long time before we will see a resulting change in bladder cancer and only small areas have so far been treated in this way.

Cancer of the Kidney

Again, the potential for prevention is great and the best identified risk factor is cigarette smoking, with estimates putting the proportion of the cancer that is attributable to smoking at between 20 and 40 per cent.

Table 9
How Much Cancer is Preventable Now and in the Future

	Preventable now (percentage)	Possibly preventable in future (percentage)
Bladder	50 (smoking)	70 (smoking)
Brain	—	—
Breast	—	30 (hormonal, diet)
Cervix	80 (screening)	80 (screening, smoking)
Colorectal	30 (diet)	30 (diet)
Kidney	20–40 (smoking)	20–40 (smoking)
Liver	20–40 (alcohol)	70 (alcohol and vaccination)
Lung	90 (smoking)	95 (smoking and radon)
Melanoma	50 (sun)	50 (sun)
Ovary	40 (hormonal)	40 (hormonal)
Pancreas	13–50 (smoking)	13–50 (smoking)
Stomach	—	50 (diet)

Leukaemia and Lymphoma

These are uncommon diseases which do show considerable variation from place to place, presumably due to environmental factors such as radiation and chemicals, or even virus infections. Regrettably, we really do not know how to translate these assumptions into effective prevention at this time.

In Table 9 we have listed the cancers from Table 8 which are the big killers in Western countries together with an estimate of the percentage of each which is preventable now and the percentage of each which we believe may be preventable in future, indicating the measures that would be appropriate for this. In Table 10 we have indicated the present benefits from effective screening and made some guesses about the possible

Table 10

How Many Cancer Deaths Could be Prevented by Effective Screening

	Reduction in number of deaths by effective screening now (percentage)	Possible reduction in number of deaths by effective screening in future (percentage)
Bladder	0	? 30 (urine tests)
Brain	0	0
Breast	30 (mammography)	30
Cervix	80 (smear tests)	80
Colorectal	0	? 30 (stool tests)
Kidney	0	0
Liver	0	0
Lung	0	0
Melanoma	0	? 50 (skin examinations)
Ovary	0	? 50 (blood and ultrasound)
Stomach	0	? 30 (X-rays and gastroscopy)

future benefits from effective screening. Again, the message is quite clear. Many, if not most, cancer deaths are due to known causes and can be prevented either by modifying the environment individually or for the community or by proper application of screening.

15
Practical Advice

The message, if you want to reduce the risk of cancer as much as possible, is quite clear:

1. **Don't smoke.**

2. **Don't smoke.**

3. **Don't smoke.**

4. **If you drink alcohol, do so in moderation.**

5. **Eat at least some fruit and vegetables and avoid a diet full of fatty foods. Most people should increase the fibre in their diet.**

6. **Avoid sunburn, particularly if you are an office worker and have a risky skin.**

7. **Take up breast and cervix screening throughout life at the recommended intervals.**

8. **Obey the Health and Safety Regulations at work.**

9. **Take some exercise.**

THE EUROPEAN CODE

Following the Europe against Cancer campaign, an anti-cancer code was developed; the main recommendations are as follows:

Firm Guidelines

- Smoking is the greatest risk factor of all – smokers stop as quickly as possible!

- Go easy on the alcohol.

- Avoid being overweight.

- Take care in the sun.

- Observe the Health and Safety regulations at work.

General Guidelines

- Cut down on fatty food.

- Eat plenty of fresh fruit and vegetables and other foods containing fibre.

- See your doctor if there is any unexplained change in your normal state of health which lasts more than two weeks.

Women

- Have a regular cervical smear test. Examine your breasts monthly (women over the age of fifty should be screened by mammography at regular intervals).

16

What Does the Future Hold?

Most people would be a little more prepared to follow the guidelines that we are promoting in this book if they were sure that there would be a real benefit and that the guidelines were not just vague advice based on scientific guesswork. In fact, there is quite a good way of reading the future in cancer. Clearly, if you look at current trends, such as the increase in incidence of malignant melanoma, they can give important pointers for the future, but we can be a bit more accurate about this. The opportunity comes from studying the trends of the incidence and death rate of cancers in different age groups. Most common cancers occur in people in their sixties and seventies or older. However, there have always been an unfortunate few who get these cancers earlier in life. For some reason they are either in a special risk category or they are in some way predisposed to get the cancers. (The reasons why they get the cancers are not important to the present argument.) They represent the first indication of a changing trend in a population because they are the ones to whom things happen after the shortest period of exposure. Since the rest of the population are also exposed to similar changes, the trends that occur in the younger patients with common cancers are likely to predict the things that will happen to the older people later on.

This is a very important argument in allowing us to read the probable future pattern for cancer. Let us consider the case of lung cancer, taking the example of a father and son. Thirty years ago, the incidence of lung cancer at the age of sixty (the father) was about 100 in 100,000 and at the age of thirty (the son) was about 10 in 100,000. These figures are rounded up

Table 11

	1950	1965	1980	1995	2010
Father (60)	100	100	100	[100]	[50]
Son (30)	10	10	5	↓?	↓?

These figures are estimates of the actual number of people who get lung cancer in each age group (at about thirty or at about sixty). The incidence in the younger group is about one tenth of that in the older group in 1950. Some changes occur between 1965 and 1980 which reduce the incidence first in the young people (by 50 per cent). This change will not work through in the older people until this age group are in their sixties, i.e. thirty years later. However, we do expect to see the changes then and can expect improvements.

for ease of argument but are not far off the actual figures. Now, thirty years later, when the son reaches the age of sixty his risk has gone up to 100 in 100,000 simply as a result of getting older. So far the figures we have quoted are the results of actual observations.

The next question is what is the actual risk of a thirty-year-old at the present time? The result is interesting. His chance of getting lung cancer at the age of thirty has now fallen substantially and is round about 5 in 100,000. He will keep that differential relative to earlier generations as he gets older. This means that when he is sixty years old his chance of getting lung cancer should be 50 in 100,000. This last figure is a forward projection, but trends and experience to date suggest that it will be reliable.

We have set these figures out in Table 11 to try to make it easier to understand this very important argument.

If the trends in young people are predictive of the future then this is very useful. The actual reduction of cancers in people between the ages of twenty and forty will not have a big impact on the overall figure because, in that age range, cancer is fortunately quite rare. However, it predicts what will happen in the older age group in the future, and in that age group cancers

Table 12
Mortality from Cancers in 1950s and Late 1980s Compared
(1950s = 100)

Type of cancer	Men	Women
Bladder	48	45
Bowel	49	36
Brain and CNS	67	60
Breast	—	103
Cervix	—	117
Hodgkin's disease	46	64
Larynx	50	25
Leukaemia	90	81
Liver	138	163
Lung	37	88
Melanoma	250	177
Mesothelioma	210	131
Non-Hodgkin's lymphoma	126	127
Ovary	—	71
Stomach	26	25
Testes	61	—

These figures show the mortality from each cancer in the late 1980s compared to that in the 1950s in the age group 20–44 years. The figure of 100 represents the baseline in the 1950s. The figures predict future trends and most are encouraging (bladder, bowel, lung, stomach cancers, for example, are below the figure of 100), but there are worries (liver, melanoma due to sunburn, mesothelioma due to asbestos, lymphoma). Most changes can be explained by the cancers reducing in occurrence, but some reductions in death are due to better treatments (Hodgkin's disease, leukaemia, testicular cancer). Breast cancer is not changing much and may show a small increase.

are much more common. It represents a way of reading the future of cancer patterns.

What does the future hold? In Table 12 we list the mortality from certain common cancers in people aged twenty to forty-four now compared to that in the 1950s, and in Figure 21 we show the differences between age groups for lung cancer in Yorkshire, our own region in England.

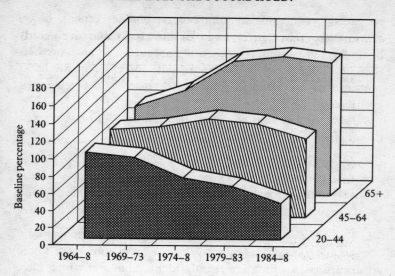

Figure 21 Incidence in Yorkshire of lung cancer in males.

The graph at the front shows the falling incidence of lung cancer in young men in Yorkshire. The trend in middle age is just beginning to be downwards. The older age group have a steady incidence but it should start decreasing soon. These figures are percentages. In actual numbers, the sixty-five-year-olds are much more important (10×) and this is the age group that determines the overall picture in the community. This means that we would not expect people to have noticed any improvement yet.

Some impressive reductions are clear, particularly for lung cancer, bowel cancer, bladder cancer and ovarian cancer. There has not been much change for breast cancer. There have been some worrying increases for malignant melanoma, cancer of the cervix, sarcomas, lymphomas and mesothelioma. These figures suggest that in future, in the United Kingdom, we will see steady reductions in lung cancer, bladder cancer, bowel cancer and ovarian cancer, and that those reductions are already being brought about by existing measures. It also predicts that, as things stand, we can anticipate increases in the other cancers that are listed as showing increases in the young age group now.

What does this kind of crystal ball tell us? We believe a few things emerge very clearly:

Environmental changes are already reducing important cancers and will continue to do so in future. These reductions are probably due to measures like low-tar cigarettes, Health and Safety regulations at work and perhaps dietary changes.

The introduction of preventive measures and environmental changes are effective and should be pursued and reinforced. There are future risks which are readily identifiable and which have already been touched on elsewhere in this book. In particular, we refer to sunburn and asbestos. Some future risks such as those involving sarcomas and lymphomas are not understood and the best guess at present might be that such cancers are caused by chemical exposure in the environment to substances such as pesticides.

The trends are good in the United Kingdom but worrying else-where. In the figure opposite we show trends for men in the age group twenty to forty-four in a range of European countries. The best data from Eastern Europe is from Hungary and this is alarming. The crystal ball there suggests increases in cancers in the next few decades compared to the prediction of reductions in Western Europe. We can only speculate why this should be. It seems likely to be related to smoking patterns and environmental, perhaps workplace, exposures.

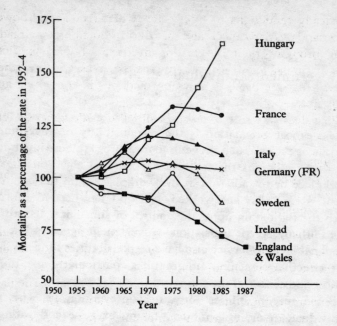

Figure 22 Trends in mortality from cancer in men aged from twenty to forty-four across Europe.

The graph reflects future trends in older people, with alarming implications in Eastern Europe.

(From Doll, R., 'Are we winning the fight against cancer? An epidemiological assessment', *European Journal of Cancer*, 1990.)

17

Government, Individuals and the National Health Service

Some cancer prevention is the responsibility of government and its agencies. Such preventive measures are best illustrated by the regulations that control exposure to chemicals in the workplace or to radiation in the workplace or in the environment. Regulation has worked well and has been reinforced with the tightening up of the control of substances hazardous to health by recent legislation. Government agencies like the National Health Service also have responsibilities for establishing effective screening programmes, particularly for breast cancer and cancer of the cervix.

Some responsibilities for cancer prevention lie with the individual. Avoiding sunburn, taking exercise and eating a healthy diet are perhaps the best examples. Identifying your own cancer risk might also be something which you should undertake in consultation with your physician. We have already given some immediate advice of this kind in this book.

Some areas of cancer prevention are the subject of dispute. The most important is the control of tobacco. Individuals clearly do have this matter in their own hands and can stop smoking. However, it is in the hands of government to take measures which make it easier for them. Does this interfere with personal liberty? This seems a pretty weak argument. Government takes it upon itself to enforce driving regulations in order to limit accidents. It does not seem unreasonable for government to introduce regulations to make it more difficult to smoke and easier not to smoke. Increasingly, regulations are restricting smoking in public places, and this is helpful. For many people in the health-care field, any action taken by governments on tobacco advertising and tobacco taxation would be taken as real evidence of their commitment to the prevention of common diseases like lung cancer and bladder cancer. In this area, individuals hold responsibility but the government can help.

Recently, for the first time in the United Kingdom, the government has introduced a document that leads towards a strategic plan for health care. This document, *The Health of the Nation*, if acted on effectively, could produce a constructive and forward-looking approach to many aspects of health care, and could be particularly relevant to the problem of cancer.

The focus of the document is upon the reduction in smoking and the future implementation of effective screening for breast cancer and cervical cancer. The ideas expressed in this book are familiar to those who are responsible for developing and implementing health strategy in the United Kingdom. It is to be hoped that the good start made in *The Health of the Nation* is followed with extensions to targets other than smoking and screening, and that we will be encouraged to develop and exploit the knowledge that we have about cancer, its causes and its prevention.

Perhaps we should start with children. The new national curriculum offers the possibility for health education across several subjects. Surveys have suggested that two thirds of secondary-school pupils are interested in the problem of cancer and would watch television programmes on this subject. They seem to be receptive, and it is perhaps especially at this age that the sort of advice which we have given in this book can be fully effective. The risk associated with smoking is an easy, straightforward and readily identifiable educational topic, but the many other recommendations which we have put forward can also be introduced readily into education at school and in the home.

Cancer is not some form of divine retribution. It is not a 'punishment' for a particular lifestyle. It is a group of diseases with biological causes which may be triggered by the way in which we lead our lives. We have a growing understanding of the features of our lifestyles which are implicated in cancer. We may, if we wish, choose to use this knowledge to reduce the risks.

Index

additives, 90, 96, 114–15, 117
aflatoxin, 90, 114, 117, 226
Africa, 59, 199–200, 202, 225–6
AIDS, 57, 59, 152, 163–5, 200
alcohol, 43–4, 48, 58, 115–17,
  221, 225–33 *passim*
Alexander, Freda, 46
alternative medicine, 86, 106
American blacks, 53
American Indians, 53
animal fats, *see* dietary fat
apple brandy, 116
asbestos
  as an environmental pollutant,
    59, 169, 178
  as an occupational hazard, 58,
    72, 167–9, 175, 191
  lung cancer, links with, 169–
    70
  mesothelioma, cause of, 36,
    168–9
atomic bombs, 57, 139, 141–6
Australia
  breast cancer study in, 99
  melanoma in, 44, 124, 127–8,
    133, 137, 227

basal cell cancer, 122–3
beer, 116–17
Belgium, 39
beta carotene, 73–4, 93, 107–14,
  117, 119
betel-nut, 111, 115

bladder cancer, 4, 11, 39, 42
  links with smoking, 55, 75, 229
  links with schistosomiasis, 218,
    229
  occupational links with, 167
bone cancer, 36, 183
bowel cancer, *see* colorectal
  cancer
Bradford Hill, Sir Austen, 65
brain cancer, 10–11, 42–3, 183,
  191
bran, 105, 119
breast cancer, 153–60, 183
  breast examination, 216, 233
  dietary fat links, 37–8, 55, 95–
    6, 98–103, 117
  growth and spread of, 9, 11,
    208
  incidence of, 39, 42, 45, 48,
    52, 227–8, 237
  obesity links, 115
  psychological factors in, 193–5
  risk rates for, 157, 184–5
  screening for, 207–8, 214–16
  socio-economic links, 30, 54,
    153, 174, 190–92
  treatment of, 4, 6, 153, 155,
    160, 214
British Journal of Cancer, 46, 147
Burkitt, Denis, 103, 199

CA 125, 218
cadmium, 72, 177

California, 52, 228
Canada, 99, 211
Cancer Mortality by Occupational and Social Class, 190
carbohydrates (*see also* starch), 88–92
carcinogens, 24–5, 68, 70, 189
Caribbean, 59, 201
Cartwright, Ray, 46, 147
case-control studies, 33, 69, 99–104 *passim*, 109, 156–7, 215
cellular differentiation, 8, 16, 19, 22
cellular proliferation, 8, 16, 19–22
cervix, cancer of the, 42, 113, 200–203, 228, 237
  and sexual activity, 59, 161–3
  cervical smear tests, 161–2, 208, 210–14
  smoking links, 55, 75, 201
  socio-economic links, 54, 190
Charlton, Ann, 79
chemicals, 58, 167, 170–73, 175–8, 191, 230
  formed in cooking, 90
chemotherapy, 4–5, 60, 64
Chernobyl, 139
childhood cancer, 6–7, 46, 133, 146–8, 180
children and smoking, 78–9, 241
chimney-sweeps, 28, 36, 58
China, 113, 200, 202
Chinese people, 45, 53, 59, 71
Christmas Island, 143–6
chrome, 72, 177
cigarettes, *see* smoking
cirrhosis of the liver, 116, 199
coal smoke, 73
cohort studies, 32–3, 59, 69, 94, 99–101, 110

coke industry, 72
colorectal cancer, 4, 19, 217
  and diet, 55, 87, 102–6, 117
  and exercise, 174–5
  genetic susceptibility to, 24, 185–6
  incidence of, 39, 42, 45, 48, 87, 225, 237–8
contraceptive pill, *see* oral contraceptives
cooking, 96, 114–15
  with a wok, 71
Cornwall, 73
COSHH (control of substances hazardous to health), 167
Crick, Francis, 12
curability of cancer, 4–7, 11, 64, 124, 134, 203–5, 214–15

Denmark, 31, 39, 104, 173, 211–12
Derbyshire, 73
Devon, 73
diet and cancer, 55–6, 73, 85–8, 95–6, 118–20, 221–2, 227–8, 232–3
dietary fat, 37, 55, 89, 92, 95–103, 117
dietary fibre, 55, 89, 95, 103–5, 117
DNA, 12–16, 180, 183–4
  and cancer of the cervix, 201
  damage to, 19, 24, 60, 72, 90, 114, 123, 139
  protection of, 108
Doll, Sir Richard, 65, 70, 88, 115, 168, 221–2
double helix, 12–14
drinking water, 3, 178–9
drug abuse, 59

drugs, *see* chemotherapy
dysplasia, 201
dysplastic naevi, 130, 183

Eastern Europe, 58, 166, 173, 238
Egypt, 218, 229
electromagnetic fields, 147
England and Wales, 31, 46, 48, 104, 146
environment, 24–5, 60, 140–43, 151, 189
  environmental pollution, 58–9, 72–3, 114, 166, 169, 176–9
environmental agents causing cancer, 171
epidemiology, the science of, 27–37, 54, 66
Epstein–Barr virus, 45, 59, 199–202
Europe against Cancer campaign, 38, 81–2
European Community, 30–31, 38–44, 48, 81–3
Euroscan, 113
exercise, 174–5, 232

familial polyposis coli, 24, 183, 185
fibre, *see* dietary fibre
Filipinos, 53
Finland, 104, 113, 211–12, 227
fish, 88, 98, 103, 114
France, 39, 43, 48, 82, 104, 116, 225
fruit, 56, 82, 93, 110, 118–19, 232–3

gall bladder, cancer of, 42–3, 115
gas industry, 72

genes (*see also* DNA), 13–25, 180, 186–7
genetic susceptibility, 23–4, 60–61, 74, 130, 133, 160, 180–87
Germany, 43, 82, 104
government, role in preventing cancer, 80–81, 86, 132, 151, 172, 240–41
Greece, 31, 39, 43, 82–3
Greer, Stephen, 194
growth of cancers, 9–11, 17, 202–3
gullet, cancer of, *see* oesophagus
gynaecological cancers, *see* cancer of the ovary and uterus

Hawaii, 45, 52–3, 71
head and neck cancer, 6, 111–13, 174, 191
Health and Safety Regulations (*see also* COSHH), 232–3
hepatitis B virus, 59, 198–9, 201, 226
herpes simplex virus, 162
Hill, Michael, 87
Hispanics, 53
Hodgkin's disease, 6, 11, 42–3, 190–91
Hong Kong, 45, 71
hormones, 55–6, 60, 152–61, 228
HRT, 157–8, 161
human papilloma virus, 57, 163, 200–202, 228
hydrocarbon, 72

Iceland, 211–12
identical twins, 74
India, 45
infections and cancer, *see* viruses

inherited cancers, 23–4, 61, 74, 180–85

International Agency for Research on Cancer, 38, 43–4, 70, 75, 170–71, 177, 190, 224

intervention studies, 33–5, 74, 94, 99–100, 110–13

invasion of cancer, 9–11, 17

Iraq, 229

Ireland, 39

Italy, 43, 82, 215

Japan, 44–5, 59, 98, 109, 201, 218–19, 225

Japanese immigrants, 52–3, 98, 228

Kaposi's sarcoma, 163

kidney cancer, 4, 55, 75, 229

Kuwait, 225

Lane, David, 23

larynx, cancer of, 42–4, 55, 75

leukaemia, 6, 60, 75, 175, 197, 201

in childhood, 146–7

incidence of, 42–3, 46, 59, 145–6

links with electromagnetic fields, 147–8

links with nuclear radiation, 46, 57, 141–7

preventability of, 230

Li–Fraumeni cancer family syndrome, 183

Linge, Elspeth, 173

lip, cancer of, 28, 42–3, 75, 174

liver cancer

incidence of, 30, 42, 174

links with alcohol, 43, 58, 115–17

links with Hepatitis B virus, 59, 164, 198–9, 202, 226

preventability of, 226

lung cancer, 7, 10, 19, 172–4, 177–8, 194

and asbestos, 72, 169–70

and atmospheric pollution, 72

and diet, 73–4

epidemic, 64–5, 84

and genes, 74

incidence of, 39, 42–3, 45–8, 185, 234–8

and income, 54, 190–91

in non-smokers, 68, 70, 77

and nuclear bombs, 145

and occupation, 72, 174

preventability of, 68, 108–13, 172–3, 227

and radon, 141, 149–50

and smoking, 27, 43, 55, 63–70, 72–5, 101, 174, 221, 227

and wok cookery, 71

Luxembourg, 31, 39

lymphoma, 42–3, 46, 60, 163, 182, 199–200, 230, 237–8

Malawi, 229

mammography, 159–60, 215–16, 233

meat, 55, 88, 90, 94–5, 102–3, 114, 117–18

medical scans, 140

melanocytes, 121

melanoma, 121

curability of, 124, 134

genetic susceptibility and skin type, 43–5, 53, 61, 123, 127–30 passim

incidence of, 42–4, 52–3, 124–7, 131, 174, 237
and ozone depletion, 122, 130–31
preventability of, 131–8, 227
and ultraviolet radiation, 58, 122, 127–8, 131–3
menopause, 56, 154, 157–9, 161
menstruation, 54, 153–4, 158
mesothelioma, 36, 167–9, 174, 237
metaplasia, 111
metastasis, 6, 9–11, 204
microbe contaminants, 90
Middle East, 45
molecular biology, 12–25
moles, 121, 129–30, 132–5
Mormons, 104
mouth cancer, 42–3, 55, 75, 111, 115–16, 225
mutagens, 24, 72, 90
myeloma, 42–3, 145–6, 167

nasopharyngeal cancer, 28, 45, 55, 200
National Health Service, 240
National Radiation Protection Board, 145, 150–51
Netherlands, 39, 43, 215
New Zealand, 225
nickel, 72, 167, 177
nicotine, 70, 76, 78
nicotine substitutes, 78
nitrates and nitrosamines, 114–15, 118
non-Hodgkin lymphomas, 6, 42–3
North America, 27, 30, 44, 128, 148, 169, 201, 225
Norway, 108, 211

nose, cancer of, see nasopharyngeal cancer
nuclear bombs, 141–6 passim
nuclear power, 139, 146–7, 151

obesity, 55, 91–2, 96, 115–19 passim, 233
occupational hazards, 58, 72, 141–2, 146–7, 166–76, 221–2
oesophagus (gullet), cancer of, 54–5, 75, 174, 191
and alcohol, 115–16
incidence of, 42–3, 48
oestrogen, 56, 153–61 passim
oncogenes, 18–25, 198, 200
oral contraceptives, 56, 155–7, 228
osteoporosis, 157–8
ovarian cancer, 42, 185, 190, 218–19, 237–8
and oral contraceptives, 56, 58, 157, 228
ozone layer, 122, 130–31

p53, 23
pancreatic cancer, 42, 75, 226
passive smoking, 55, 69, 72
personality, see psychological factors
pesticides, 90, 114, 167, 176–8, 238
Peto, Richard, 83, 221–2
Pike, Malcolm, 156
Pill, the, see oral contraceptives
platinum, 7
Poland, 124, 228
Polish immigrants, 98
Portugal, 31, 39, 42–3
Pott, Percival, 28, 36, 58
pregnancy, 143, 154

progesterone, 153, 158–61 *passim*
prostatic cancer, 39, 42, 45, 48, 155, 229
protein in diet, 85, 89–92 *passim*
psychological factors, 192–6

quality of life, 7, 85, 106, 194–6
Queensland, 45, 124, 227

racial variations, 52–3, 60–61
radiation, 22, 36, 57, 72–3, 139–47, 149–51, 175, 222, 230
   as electromagnetic fields, 147–8
   as ultraviolet light, 122, 131
radiotherapy, 4, 5, 63–4, 204–5
radon
   as atmospheric pollutant, 57, 73, 140–41, 144, 149–50, 177
   as occupational hazard, 57, 72, 141
rape-seed oil, 71
rectum, cancer of, *see* colorectal cancer
retinoblastoma, 23–4, 183
retinoic acid, 107–8
retro-viruses (*see also* AIDS), 198, 201
RNA, 13
Rous, Peyton, 197
Royal College of Physicians, *Smoking and the Young*, 70

safe sex, 164–5
sarcomas, 237–8
Scandinavia, 43, 73, 104, 131, 211–13
schistosomiasis, 218, 229
Scotland, 31, 48, 124–5, 215

Scottish Melanoma Group, 134
screening
   and cancer biology, 203–10
   for bladder cancer, 218
   for bowel cancer, 217, 220
   for breast cancer, 155, 207–8, 214–16, 219, 232–3
   for cervical cancer, 161–2, 192, 201, 208, 210–14, 219, 228, 232–3
   for lung cancer, 217
   for ovarian cancer, 218
   for stomach cancer, 218–19
   pitfalls, 209–10
scrotum, cancer of, 28
selenium, 93–4, 96, 113–14
Sellafield, 46, 146–7
Seventh Day Adventists, 98, 100, 104
sexual activity, 56–7, 59, 152, 162–5, 202
sexual differences, 39–43
skin cancer, *see* basal cell cancers; squamous cell cancers; melanoma
skin classification, 129
smoked foods, 114–15, 118
smoking
   addiction, 76
   and alcohol, 48, 116
   and genes, 22, 74
   and lung cancer, 27, 43, 55, 63–70, 72–5, 101, 174, 221, 227
   and other cancers, 75, 201, 221, 226, 219
   giving up, 76–8, 232–3
   government policies on, 80–83, 240–41
   socio-economic factors in, 190–92

sociological factors, 53–4, 153, 189–92
Somerset, 46
South Africa, 168
soya-bean oil, 71–2
Spain, 39, 43, 82–3, 225–6
spread of cancer, *see* metastasis
squamous cell cancer, 122–3
starch, 55, 95, 103–6
stomach cancer, 39, 42, 45, 52–5 *passim*, 75, 115, 118, 190, 194, 225
stress, *see* psychological factors
sunlight, 58, 121–8 *passim*, 130–33, 135–8, 222, 232–3
surgery, 4, 5, 10–11, 63, 161, 195
Sweden, 150, 179, 211–12, 215
Swerdlow, Tony, 46
Switzerland, 226

Taiwan, 199
Tamoxifen, 153, 155, 160, 165
testis, cancer of, 6, 11, 42, 190–91
testosterone, 155
Tobacco (*see also* smoking), 55, 80–84, 111, 115, 225
tumour suppressor genes, 22–5

ultrasound, 217–18
ultraviolet irradiation, *see* sunlight
ultraviolet sensors, 135–6
United Kingdom, 1, 6, 43, 45–6, 69, 73, 78, 104, 124–5, 143–4, 178, 241
    and breast cancer, 156–7, 160, 214
    cervical screening programme, 211–14

incidence rates in, 39, 43, 45–58, 125, 214, 227, 237–8
radiation protection in, 142, 151, 167
radon centration in, 73, 149–50
United States, 31, 53, 65, 69, 98–100, 104, 124–5, 146, 149–50, 155–6, 166, 179
    and breast cancer, 99–100, 156, 160, 215, 227–8
    incidence rates in, 45, 52
    interventions studies in, 108–9, 113
    studies on effects of radon, 73, 150
uranium mining, 57, 72, 149
uterus, cancer of, 42, 52, 54–6, 115, 161

vaccinations, 202, 226, 228
vegetables, 56, 82, 92–3, 110, 118–19, 232–3
vinyl chloride, 72
viruses, 197–202, 222
    Epstein–Barr virus, 45, 59, 199–200
    herpes simplex, 162
    human papilloma, 57, 163, 200–201, 228
    human T lymphotrophic virus type 1, 59
    link to oncogenes, 18–22 *passim*, 59, 198
    retro-viruses (*see also* AIDS), 198, 201
vitamins and minerals, 56, 85, 92, 106, 119–20
    vitamin A and related, 73, 89, 96, 107–14, 117

vitamins and minerals—*contd*
  vitamin C, 89, 114
  vitamin E, 96, 113–14
  selenium, 93–4, 96, 113–14

Wald, Nicholas, 69–70
Watson, James, 12
Wertheimer and Leeper, 147–8
Western Europe, 27, 58, 67, 104,
  124–5, 155, 166, 169, 225,
  238
white-skinned people, 53, 61, 123,
  129, 132, 227

wine (*see also* alcohol), 116
woks, 71
womb, *see* uterus
workplace risks, *see* occupational
  hazards
World Health Organization, 83,
  210

X-rays, 9, 57, 140, 143, 151,
  159–60, 215–17

Yorkshire, 236–7

Discover more about our forthcoming books through Penguin's FREE newspaper...

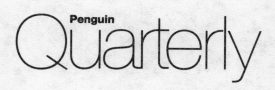

Penguin **Quarterly**

It's packed with:

- exciting features
- author interviews
- previews & reviews
- books from your favourite films & TV series
- exclusive competitions & much, much more...

Write off for your free copy today to:
Dept JC
Penguin Books Ltd
FREEPOST
West Drayton
Middlesex
UB7 0BR
NO STAMP REQUIRED

READ MORE IN PENGUIN

In every corner of the world, on every subject under the sun, Penguin represents quality and variety – the very best in publishing today.

For complete information about books available from Penguin – including Puffins, Penguin Classics and Arkana – and how to order them, write to us at the appropriate address below. Please note that for copyright reasons the selection of books varies from country to country.

In the United Kingdom: Please write to *Dept. JC, Penguin Books Ltd, FREEPOST, West Drayton, Middlesex UB7 OBR*

If you have any difficulty in obtaining a title, please send your order with the correct money, plus ten per cent for postage and packaging, to *PO Box No. 11, West Drayton, Middlesex UB7 OBR*

In the United States: Please write to *Penguin USA Inc., 375 Hudson Street, New York, NY 10014*

In Canada: Please write to *Penguin Books Canada Ltd, 10 Alcorn Avenue, Suite 300, Toronto, Ontario M4V 3B2*

In Australia: Please write to *Penguin Books Australia Ltd, 487 Maroondah Highway, Ringwood, Victoria 3134*

In New Zealand: Please write to *Penguin Books (NZ) Ltd, 182–190 Wairau Road, Private Bag, Takapuna, Auckland 9*

In India: Please write to *Penguin Books India Pvt Ltd, 706 Eros Apartments, 56 Nehru Place, New Delhi 110 019*

In the Netherlands: Please write to *Penguin Books Netherlands B.V., Keizersgracht 231 NL–1016 DV Amsterdam*

In Germany: Please write to *Penguin Books Deutschland GmbH, Friedrichstrasse 10–12, W–6000 Frankfurt/Main 1*

In Spain: Please write to *Penguin Books S. A., C. San Bernardo 117–6° E–28015 Madrid*

In Italy: Please write to *Penguin Italia s.r.l., Via Felice Casati 20, I–20124 Milano*

In France: Please write to *Penguin France S. A., 17 rue Lejeune, F–31000 Toulouse*

In Japan: Please write to *Penguin Books Japan, Ishikiribashi Building, 2–5–4, Suido, Tokyo 112*

In Greece: Please write to *Penguin Hellas Ltd, Dimocritou 3, GR–106 71 Athens*

In South Africa: Please write to *Longman Penguin Southern Africa (Pty) Ltd, Private Bag X08, Bertsham 2013*

READ MORE IN PENGUIN

A SELECTION OF HEALTH BOOKS

The Kind Food Guide   Audrey Eyton

Audrey Eyton's all-time bestselling *The F-Plan Diet* turned the nation on to fibre-rich food. Now, as the tide turns against factory farming, she provides the guide destined to bring in a new era of eating.

Baby and Child   Penelope Leach

A beautifully illustrated and comprehensive handbook on the first five years of life. 'It stands head and shoulders above anything else available at the moment' – Mary Kenny in the *Spectator*

Woman's Experience of Sex   Sheila Kitzinger

Fully illustrated with photographs and line drawings, this book explores the riches of women's sexuality at every stage of life. 'A book which any mother could confidently pass on to her daughter – and her partner too' – *Sunday Times*

A Guide to Common Illnesses   Dr Ruth Lever

The complete, up-to-date guide to common complaints and their treatment, from causes and symptoms to cures, explaining both orthodox and complementary approaches.

Living with Alzheimer's Disease and Similar Conditions
Dr Gordon Wilcock

This complete and compassionate self-help guide is designed for families and carers (professional or otherwise) faced with the 'living bereavement' of dementia.

Living with Stress
Cary L. Cooper, Rachel D. Cooper and Lynn H. Eaker

Stress leads to more stress, and the authors of this helpful book show why low levels of stress are desirable and how best we can achieve them in today's world. Looking at those most vulnerable, they demonstrate ways of breaking the vicious circle that can ruin lives.

READ MORE IN PENGUIN

A SELECTION OF HEALTH BOOKS

Living with Asthma and Hay Fever   John Donaldson

For the first time, there are now medicines that can prevent asthma attacks from taking place. Based on up-to-date research, this book shows how the majority of sufferers can beat asthma and hay fever to lead full and active lives.

Anorexia Nervosa   R. L. Palmer

Lucid and sympathetic guidance for those who suffer from this disturbing illness and their families and professional helpers, given with a clarity and compassion that will make anorexia more understandable and consequently less frightening for everyone involved.

Medical Treatments: Benefits and Risks   Peter Parish

The ultimate reference guide to the drug treatments available today – from over-the-counter remedies to drugs given under close medical supervision – for every common disease or complaint from acne to worms.

Pregnancy and Childbirth   Sheila Kitzinger
Revised Edition

A complete and up-to-date guide to physical and emotional preparation for pregnancy – a must for all prospective parents.

Miscarriage   Ann Oakley, Ann McPherson and Helen Roberts

One million women worldwide become pregnant every day. At least half of these pregnancies end in miscarriage or stillbirth. But each miscarriage is the loss of a potential baby, and that loss can be painful to adjust to. Here is sympathetic support and up-to-date information on one of the commonest areas of women's reproductive experience.

The Parents' A-Z   Penelope Leach

For anyone with children of 6 months, 6 years or 16 years, this guide to all the little problems in their health, growth and happiness will prove reassuring and helpful.

READ MORE IN PENGUIN

A SELECTION OF HEALTH BOOKS

When a Woman's Body Says No to Sex Linda Valins

Vaginismus – an involuntary spasm of the vaginal muscles that prevents penetration – has been discussed so little that many women who suffer from it don't recognize their condition by its name. Linda Valins's practical and compassionate guide will liberate these women from their fears and sense of isolation and help them find the right form of therapy.

Medicine The Self-Help Guide
Professor Michael Orme and Dr Susanna Grahame-Jones

A new kind of home doctor – with an entirely new approach. With a unique emphasis on self-management, *Medicine* takes an active approach to drugs, showing how to maximize their benefits, speed up recovery and minimize dosages through self-help and non-drug alternatives.

Defeating Depression Tony Lake

Counselling, medication, and the support of friends can all provide invaluable help in relieving depression. But if we are to combat it once and for all, we must face up to perhaps painful truths about our past and take the first steps forward that can eventually transform our lives. This lucid and sensitive book shows us how.

Freedom and Choice in Childbirth Sheila Kitzinger

Undogmatic, honest and compassionate, Sheila Kitzinger's book raises searching questions about the kind of care offered to the pregnant woman – and will help her make decisions and communicate effectively about the kind of birth experience she desires.

Care of the Dying Richard Lamerton

It is never true that 'nothing more can be done' for the dying. This book shows us how to face death without pain, with humanity, with dignity and in peace.